© Copyright (09-01-2023) by Kalil L

This document is geared towards providing exact and reliable information in regards to the topic and issue covered. The publication is sold with the idea that the publisher is not required to render accounting, officially permitted, or otherwise, qualified services. If advice is necessary, legal or professional, a practiced individual in the profession should be ordered.
- From a Declaration of Principles which was accepted and approved equally by a Committee of the American Bar Association and a Committee of Publishers and Associations.
In no way is it legal to reproduce, duplicate, or transmit any part of this document in either electronic means or in printed format. Recording of this publication is strictly prohibited and any storage of this document is not allowed unless with written permission from the publisher. All rights reserved.
The information provided herein is stated to be truthful and consistent, in that any liability, in terms of inattention or otherwise, by any usage or abuse of any policies, processes, or directions contained within is the solitary and utter responsibility of the recipient reader. Under no circumstances will any legal responsibility or blame be held against the publisher for any reparation, damages, or monetary loss due to the information herein, either directly or indirectly.
Respective authors own all copyrights not held by the publisher.
The information herein is offered for informational purposes solely, and is universal as so. The presentation of the information is without contract or any type of guarantee assurance.
The trademarks that are used are without any consent, and the publication of the trademark is without permission or backing by the trademark owner. All trademarks and brands within this book are for clarifying purposes only and are owned by the owners themselves, not affiliated with this document.

# PREAMBLE

## YOU DON'T HAVE TO BE GREAT TO START, BUT YOU DO HAVE TO START TO BE GREAT

Close your eyes and envision a life where you feel physically fit, where you can purchase any clothes without worrying about your size, where walking a few hundred yards doesn't leave you sweaty and out of breath, where you radiate a natural glow and feel attractive, where others notice and compliment your appearance. This can be your reality with the ABCS of FAT LOSS. Indeed, this book provides all the necessary knowledge and guidance to not only achieve your fitness goals but also maintain them over time.

Inside this book, you'll discover more than just tips and tricks for achieving and maintaining fitness. Its primary focus is to educate you about how your body works, empowering you to take control and truly understand it. Armed with this knowledge, you'll be able to reclaim ownership of your body and make informed decisions about how to treat it right.

But first, we must understand a few things, and we have to ask ourselves a few questions.

Why are you fat? What drove you to this situation? What is keeping you fat and unhealthy? That's the three questions we are going to answer DEEPLY and <u>MOST IMPORTANTLY DEFINITELY</u> through this book.

Now, let's begin our exploration into the vast sea of body knowledge without any delay. Remember, the journey toward a healthier you, doesn't require greatness from the start, but it does necessitate that you take that first step toward making positive changes. Only by beginning can you hope to achieve greatness.

## I WISH I KNEW THAT A LONG TIME AGO

When I see a person with excess fat, the only thing that I see is a person with a DISRUPTED BRAIN.

THAT'S IT. AS SIMPLE AS THAT. NOTHING MORE NOTHING LESS. That could seem a little bit simplistic, or inexact, but it is a simple truth.

It's important to understand that anything that throws off your brain's equilibrium and overall well-being will also have a negative impact on your body weight. This is an immutable law that you must prioritize above all else. This book aims to provide you with all the information you need to get your brain back on track. Although the process may be challenging, if you gradually rewire your brain, your body weight will naturally and automatically fall into place. However, there's a catch: the law works in both directions. If your brain becomes unbalanced again, your body weight will follow suit. But fear not, the ABCS of FAT LOSS is here to guide you through the errors that have caused your brain to become unbalanced and all the steps you must take to regain control of your body fat.

In the following chapters, we are going to cover ALL THE MECHANISM that will help you understand, why you have been accumulating so much fat during the last months/years/decades, and most importantly, the mechanism that will show you how to LOSE it for good this time, and never get fat again.

I want to emphasize that the information contained in this book is just that - information. It's up to you to act and implement this information into your life. If you fail to make the necessary adjustments, then I regret to say that your health and life will remain unchanged. However, if you do take action and apply the knowledge provided, I can confidently promise you that you'll experience remarkable results in a surprisingly short amount of time. Best of all, you won't feel fatigued or overwhelmed in the process.

# INTRODUCTION

In the pursuit of health and vitality, few journeys are as universal and transformative as the quest to shed unwanted fat. Whether you're starting your journey towards a healthier you or looking to fine-tune your existing approach, "The ABCs of Fat Loss" is your comprehensive guide, designed to demystify the complexities of weight management.

Fat loss isn't just about aesthetics; it's about reclaiming your energy, enhancing your well-being, and maximizing your potential. It's about unlocking the door to a more vibrant and fulfilling life.

In this book, we will embark on a journey together, exploring the fundamental principles, strategies, and insights that underpin effective fat loss. From the science behind metabolism to the psychology of cravings, from the importance of nutrition to the power of exercise, we'll delve into the ABCs of Fat Loss to equip you with the knowledge and tools you need to succeed.

But this book isn't just about numbers on a scale or counting calories. It's about understanding your body, embracing sustainable habits, and fostering a positive relationship with food and fitness. It's about making informed choices that empower you to take control of your health and well-being.

We'll navigate the myths and misconceptions surrounding fat loss, replacing them with evidence-based information that empowers you to make choices that align with your unique goals and values. "The ABCs of Fat Loss" isn't a one-size-fits-all solution; it's a flexible framework that can be tailored to your individual needs and preferences.

Throughout this journey, we'll also explore the often-overlooked but vital role of sleep, stress management, and mindfulness in your fat loss equation. These components are the unsung heroes of your journey, and understanding their significance is key to long-term success.

Each chapter of this book will dive deep into a different aspect of fat loss, providing practical tips, actionable advice, and real-world examples to help you navigate the challenges and triumphs of your journey. You'll discover how to set realistic goals, create sustainable habits, and overcome common obstacles that can hinder your progress.

"The ABCs of Fat Loss" isn't a quick fix or a crash diet; it's a holistic approach to improving your health and well-being that extends beyond fat loss. It's about reclaiming control of your body, your choices, and your future.

So, whether you're just beginning your journey or seeking to refine your existing strategies, join me as we embark on this enlightening and empowering exploration of fat loss. Together, we'll learn, grow, and transform, one letter at a time, as we navigate the ABCs of fat loss.

## A FEW NUMBERS

According to the World Health Organization:

- The risk of premature death increases as BMI increases. According to a study published in JAMA in 2016, the risk of premature death was lowest in people with a BMI between 20 and 24.9. Compared with this group, the risk of premature death was 31% higher in people with a BMI between 25 and 29.9, 58% higher in people with a BMI between 30 and 34.9, and 88% higher in people with a BMI of 35 or higher.
- Obesity has tripled since 1975.
- In 2016, more than 1.9 billion adults, 18 years and older, were overweight. 650 million were obese in 2016 and 800 million by 2021.
- 39% of adults aged 18 years and over were overweight in 2016, and 13% were obese.
- Most of the world's population lives in countries where overweight and obesity kills more people than underweight.

- 39 million children under the age of 5 were overweight or obese in 2020.
- Over 340 million children and adolescents aged 5-19 were overweight or obese in 2016.
- By 2030, an estimated 20% of the world's population will be obese. **AN ESTIMATED 50% OF THE US POPULATION WILL BE OBESE.**
- By 2050, 60 to 80 % of adults living in Western countries are expected to be obese.
- For persons with severe obesity (BMI ≥40), life expectancy is reduced by as much as 20 years in men.
- **IN 2020 44% of Americans were obese.**
- **AROUND 2.8 MILLION PEOPLE DIE EACH YEAR BECAUSE OF OBESITY.**
- **50 million people die each year from obesity-related causes.**
- **Any death before 120 years is considered an EARLY DEATH.**
- **OBESITY IS PREVENTABLE.**

These statistics are truly alarming, and unfortunately, they are on the rise with no clear solution in sight. The fact that obesity is preventable makes the situation even more devastating. It's difficult to fathom how anyone could accept living an unhealthy lifestyle and risk dying prematurely, missing out on the opportunity to reach their full potential. It's simply madness.

The answer to this question is quite simple - when your mind lacks willpower and your body lacks energy, how can you possibly make any meaningful changes? Adding to this predicament is the fact that our education system provides very little information about our bodies, health, lifestyle, and nutrition. Despite attending school for up to 15 years or more, we are left with minimal knowledge on these important topics. This book aims to change that. The ABCs of FAT LOSS will equip you with all the information and tools necessary to achieve your desired body goals and unlock your full potential.

## CLEAR ACHIEVABLE GOALS

Congratulations on your decision to shed the excess fat you've accumulated over the years and regain your health and take control of your life. It's a significant step, and you should be proud of yourself. Now, it's time to set your goals and write them down. Studies have demonstrated that the more specific you are in setting your goals, the higher the likelihood of achieving them. Therefore, it's crucial to establish your goals for each day, week, month, 2 months, 6 months, and 1 year. What are your objectives in each of these timeframes? Be clear and specific, and you'll be on your way to success.

Set them very carefully and very precisely regarding what is your status in life in general. For instance, a 20-year-old student before the summer will not have the same goal as a 40 years young woman (yes 40 years is very young) with a job, two children, and a household to take care of.

## WARNING

Rest assured that all the information contained in this book is backed by scientific research and expert medical opinions. Not a single piece of information in this book will be disputed by any reputable doctor on the planet. You can trust that the advice provided in this book is accurate, reliable, and evidence-based.

**However, before beginning any physical activity, it's crucial to consult not just one, but multiple doctors and discuss your condition. It's important to start slow and gradually build up intensity, as working out at a high level can be dangerous to anyone if not approached with caution. It's essential to be mindful of your present physical state and tailor your fitness routine accordingly. Keep in mind that getting healthy is not a sprint, but rather a marathon - so take your time, stay committed, and don't rush the process.**

# THE ALPHABET OF FAT LOSS AND HEALTH

# A

## A for ACCOUNTABILITY

Accountability is key to successful fat loss, going beyond mere responsibility to acknowledging the results of your actions, good or bad. Strategies such as diligent food tracking, regular weigh-ins, and seeking professional advice can keep you accountable, providing motivation and focus amid challenges.

The power of accountability stems from its urgency. Being aware that your progress is monitored makes it harder to slip, with the support of others serving as a compelling motivation to adhere to your plan. A support network can also be crucial during tough times, providing guidance and reassurance that you're not alone.

Accountability encourages self-honesty, preventing self-deception about your progress or setbacks and enabling you to confront the reality, whether pleasant or not. Such honesty is a crucial step towards success.

This process involves vulnerability, openness, and trust in those you're accountable to. While it can be tough, developing such trust leads to great rewards. Having supportive, honest people, such as a coach, a group, or a friend with shared goals, is essential for effective accountability.

Another critical aspect of accountability is the willingness to accept feedback and make necessary adjustments. Defensiveness or excuses won't help you progress. True accountability involves taking ownership of your actions and their outcomes, understanding that you have the power to shape your life and the responsibility to make wise decisions aligning with your goals.

If you're struggling with fat loss, integrating accountability measures like diet tracking, regular weigh-ins, or mentorship can lead to remarkable progress, setting you on a path towards a healthier future.

## A for ACCUMULATION

Understanding that our current weight is the result of past choices can be a powerful step towards fat loss. It's often easy to blame external factors, but ultimately, our decisions about food and exercise largely dictate our weight. Acknowledging this truth transforms us from victims to active managers of our health.

Accepting our past mistakes is challenging, but doing so liberates us from guilt and shame often tied to being overweight. Instead of dwelling on past missteps or fearing substantial lifestyle changes, we can start making small, manageable improvements. Every healthier choice, like opting for a salad or going for a walk, edges us towards our goal.

Recognizing that our past decisions shape our present situation illuminates our ability to make different, healthier choices for a better future. We can't change our past, but we can influence our present and future by making decisions aligned with our values and goals. This liberates us from feeling stuck in unhealthy patterns, empowering us to forge a new path.

Changing deeply ingrained habits and embracing new ones requires patience, commitment, and bravery to face the discomfort of change. By concentrating on present choices, we can gradually shape a healthier reality. Seeing the benefits of healthier choices, such as fat loss, increased energy, or improved mood, motivates us to stay the course.

In essence, acknowledging our current state as a result of our past choices is a crucial step for sustainable fat loss. Though accepting past errors may be hard, it equips us to take charge of our health. By focusing on daily choices and slowly cultivating healthier habits, we set the stage for a healthier future. Let's let go of the past, seize the present, and embark on positive changes today.

## A for ACTION

Embarking on the path to improved health and wellness involves more than just acquiring information, like what this book provides. The real key lies in implementing the learned changes in your life. Remember, the responsibility of your health rests solely on you. Though it's tempting to seek external solutions or miracle cures, genuine change is in your hands.

Change can be daunting, and a lifestyle overhaul may seem insurmountable. However, significant results often stem from small actions. It's not about overnight transformation but steady strides towards a healthier, happier you.

Don't overlook the importance of time. Delaying action allows unhealthy habits to entrench and potentially harm you. If you don't take health matters into your hands, your life might be at stake. On a brighter note, taking charge of your health equals regaining control of your life. You'll feel energetic, healthier, and more equipped to live life to its fullest. The perfect time to start is now, and it begins with the decision to act.

Reflect on your life and health aspirations. What transformations do you seek? What immediate small steps can you take towards those goals? Remember, progress triumphs over perfection.

In conclusion, the knowledge presented in this book is merely the first step. The next is to turn this information into action, gaining control of your health and life. Now is the time to start. So, take a deep breath, decide to change, and let's embark on this journey together.

## A for ADAPTATION

After laying the groundwork for healthier habits, you'll encounter the phase of adaptation. Life's unpredictable nature might throw curveballs your way, interrupting your routine. However, it's crucial to persist with your health commitments, like maintaining a balanced diet and consistent exercise, no matter the circumstances.

Unanticipated disruptions may tempt you to neglect your health commitments, but giving in will only hamper your progress. Instead, adapt and persevere. If you can't hit the gym because of a broken car, do a home workout. If time doesn't allow you to cook healthy meals, meal prep on Sundays for the week. If you're out of nutritious groceries, research restaurants serving healthy dishes or grab some raw foods requiring no cooking.

By preparing alternative plans beforehand, you can handle surprises without compromising your health routine. Understand that situations won't always be ideal, so it's on you to make it work. Have a plan, stick to it, but be ready to modify it as needed.

The ultimate objective is to make healthy habits an integral part of your lifestyle. It's not an overnight transformation but a gradual process achieved by sustained commitment and adaptive methods. So, cherish the journey, don't be disheartened by minor setbacks, and see every day as a chance to progress towards a healthier, happier you.

## A for ADD

A common mistake people make when starting a fat loss journey is believing that they need to reduce, subtract, and diminish their food intake. However, this is a big mistake. To achieve and maintain a healthy body, it's crucial to understand your body's mechanisms and be aware of your current physical state.

Before starting a diet, it's common to feel tired and deficient in nutrients. Removing things from your diet may only worsen the situation. Instead, you should focus on re-educating your entire body by adding nutritious foods to your diet.

This is not a frustrating diet that will lead to the same unsuccessful outcomes as before. This is a life diet, the first step in a joyful process where you embrace the changes you make. Therefore, rather than focusing on what you must remove from your diet and lifestyle, concentrate on what you can add. The goal is to achieve vitality and health, and patience is essential to reach that goal.

## A for ADDICTION

Addiction and fat loss are interconnected issues that can make a healthy lifestyle challenging. Food addiction, particularly, can lead to indulgence in comfort foods, often under stress or emotional distress, and can hinder fat loss. To tackle this, identifying triggers that lead to cravings is essential, forming the basis for strategies to manage them.

Developing healthier coping mechanisms is crucial, as food often becomes a solace during stress. Options like exercise, mindfulness, or social support can help in managing emotions without resorting to food. Additionally, addressing underlying mental health issues like depression or anxiety, which can aggravate addiction and disrupt healthy eating, is vital. Professional assistance through therapy or medication can help in these cases.

Substance abuse, including alcohol, can derail fat loss efforts by increasing appetite and reducing motivation for healthy behaviors. Overcoming this requires professional help and the creation of healthy coping strategies. Moreover, the risk of relapse is real in the context of addiction and fat loss, making a supportive environment invaluable for staying on track.

Poor nutrition often accompanies addiction, so addressing nutritional deficiencies is key for overall health and better management of addiction. Additionally, factors like genetics and health conditions can influence fat loss, necessitating a holistic approach.

Strategies like Cognitive-Behavioral Therapy (CBT) and Mindfulness-Based Stress Reduction (MBSR) can be effective. CBT aids in modifying negative thought patterns and behaviors, while MBSR helps manage stress and emotions better through mindfulness.

In sum, tackling addiction is pivotal for successful fat loss. This requires a holistic approach—identifying triggers, forming healthier coping mechanisms, addressing mental health, and seeking professional aid when needed. A supportive environment can help manage relapses, and with the right tools, enduring fat loss, and improved health are attainable.

## A for ADDITIVES

Food additives are substances added to food to enhance safety, freshness, taste, texture, or appearance, according to the World Health Organization. Although some additives like salt, sugar, and sulfur dioxide have been used for centuries, many modern additives can be harmful.

Every year, we consume a significant quantity of food additives present in many manufactured products, including potato chips, soda, pre-packaged meals, fast food, and infant formula. Often, these are used to disguise poor product quality and encourage increased consumption, potentially leading to addictive patterns.

Nutritionist Corinne Gouget, in her book "Food Additives, DANGER, the essential guide not to poison yourself anymore," categorizes food additives from safe to hazardous. She suggests that only a small percentage are genuinely safe, with the rest varying from high-risk to extremely dangerous.

Food additives also influence us to consume other potentially harmful substances. For instance, after eating a salty burger and fries, our body, striving for acid-base balance, might crave sugar and water, leading us to consume sugary desserts and large sodas. This way, we end up ingesting a cocktail of potentially harmful substances, including sugar, salt, lactose, gluten, additives, sauces, and low-quality meat.

In conclusion, the widespread use of food additives can negatively impact our health. It's critical to be aware of the additives in our food and their potential health implications. Choosing healthier food options, avoiding harmful additives, and maintaining a healthy lifestyle are key to preserving our overall well-being.

## A for ADJUSTMENTS

If you're not meeting your goals and feel stuck, it's time to reassess your habits and adopt new ones. It's a common pitfall to remain in comfortable but unproductive routines, like excessive TV watching, excessive social media scrolling, or unhealthy eating.

For meaningful change and growth, you need to shift your lifestyle. Prioritize the aspects that truly matter to you, such as physical activity, family time, or nurturing a hobby. Examine your dietary habits, too. If your diet is dominated by convenient but unhealthy foods, consider making a shift towards balanced, nutritious eating. Transitioning to more wholesome foods can be challenging but it rewards with better physical health and well-being.

Also, evaluate your daily routines. If you're consistently sacrificing rest and relaxation in the pursuit of productivity, it's time to recalibrate. Prioritizing self-care activities like adequate sleep, mindfulness practices, and timely breaks can drastically improve your lifestyle.

Adopting positive changes is a continuous process requiring time, patience, and commitment. It involves steadily building new habits while releasing old ones. However, each incremental change you make brings you closer to your desired life.

If you're feeling overwhelmed and unsure where to begin, start by identifying the areas you struggle in, and make minor, sustainable changes towards your goals. Be it incorporating more physical activity in your day, practicing gratitude, or taking mindful breaths during stressful moments, each small positive change gets you nearer to the life you aspire to live.

Remember, while change is hard, it's always worthwhile. With patience, determination, and willingness to break old habits, you can attain any goal. So why not start today? Your future is filled with endless possibilities.

## A for AGENDA

Putting an organization in motion is a MUST. I repeat, putting an organization in motion is a MUST.

In life, we may have different backgrounds, financial statuses, genetics, and nationalities, but there's one thing that unites us all - we all have 24 hours in a day. The key difference between a healthy and unhealthy person, a fit person, and an overweight person, is their unwavering commitment to their well-being. No matter what happens in their day, their schedule remains the same. They know exactly what they need to do in terms of exercise, nutrition, and self-care to stay fit and healthy, and they stick to it with discipline and determination.

Thus, what you must understand is that there are 4 categories of activities to put in your daily calendar:

- 1, THE MANDATORY
- 2, THE HIGHLY RECOMMENDED
- 3, THE OPTIONAL
- 4, THE FUN ONES

How you choose to put each activity in one of those categories will change not only your body, but your mindset, your health, and your revenues. In other words, it will change your lifestyle.

Just as work, sleep, hygiene, and eating are necessary for life, fun activities like watching a game or a favorite show also play a vital role in maintaining balance. Organizing your daily activities thoughtfully can greatly enhance your overall health, energy, lifestyle, and even income. Certain activities, like healthy eating and exercise, should be mandatory and non-negotiable, except on rest days.

To optimally structure your day, it's essential to be precise and methodical. Begin by identifying your weekly tasks and categorize them into four groups: mandatory, highly recommended, optional, and fun. Mandatory tasks might include work, hygiene, and sleep, while highly recommended ones could be exercise and preparing nutritious meals. Optional tasks might be attending social gatherings or running errands, and fun activities could involve watching TV or gaming. Prioritize and schedule your tasks according to their importance and stick to your plan.

Though your calendar might seem overwhelming, by including the information of this book in your life, you'll have sufficient energy to manage your day effectively, from cooking and working out to grocery shopping. This level of organization can lead to significant improvements in your lifestyle, health, and energy.

## A for ALICAMENT (functional food)

What is alicament? It's the French contraction between **ALI**ment (food) and medi**CAMENT** (medicine).

For centuries, food has been used as a means of healing the body. By changing your diet, you cannot only shed excess fat but also promote healing within your body. Eating nutritious foods can help reduce inflammation, fight off small tumors, alleviate conditions such as osteoarthritis, back pain, and diabetes, and even improve your vision, cardiovascular health, mood, and mental state.

On the other hand, consuming unhealthy, processed foods has been linked to lethargy, illness, low energy levels, lack of motivation, and constant feelings of hunger and anger. It can also lead to a brain fog that makes it difficult to make the right decisions. Therefore, learning how to prepare fresh, seasonal vegetables can be a crucial step in promoting both physical and mental well-being.

Your diet plays a significant role in determining your overall health and vitality. It affects not only your weight but also your energy levels, mood, and overall quality of life. By making conscious choices about what you eat, you can take charge of your health and improve your overall well-being.

## A for ALKALINE VS ACIDIC

Our body's health and well-being hinge on a balance of factors, including our pH level, which marks the equilibrium between acidity and alkalinity. An overly acidic body can trigger various health problems, from inflammation and chronic pain to severe diseases like cancer, diabetes, hypertension, and even mental effects such as low motivation and brain fog.

Our diet significantly influences our body's acidity. Acidic foods like processed items, sugar, alcohol, and meats can increase body acidity, while alkaline foods, mostly fresh fruits and vegetables, help sustain a healthy pH balance.

Our body's optimal pH level lies between 7.2 and 7.4. Blood pH, ideally between 7.35 and 7.45, also plays a crucial role in managing acidity. If it falls below 7.35, severe health issues may ensue.

Fortunately, dietary and lifestyle changes can maintain a healthy pH balance. The information in this book is advocating for a diet rich in fresh fruits and vegetables, hydration, stress reduction, ample sleep, and avoiding acidic foods, effectively managing body acidity. This balance is vital for those aiming for fat loss, as an overly acidic body can slow metabolism, hindering fat loss.

In essence, understanding the impact of pH balance on our health and fat loss is key. By making the right diet and lifestyle choices, including following the information of this book and consuming alkaline foods, a healthy pH balance can be achieved, boosting metabolism and improving overall well-being.

## A for ALONE

Coming to terms with the reality of fat loss can be tough; however, it is a journey you must undertake on your own. While you might have supportive friends and family, the challenge of losing weight, the physical discomfort, the emotional stress, and missed opportunities due to excess weight, is yours to bear. But acknowledging you alone can make the necessary changes is the first step to success.

It is you who must commit to the hard work - exercise, resist unhealthy food, and make sacrifices. Not taking action can lead to severe consequences for your physical and emotional well-being. While your loved ones might be supportive, they can't do the work for you due to their own responsibilities and limitations. This is why it's vital to have a sincere conversation with yourself, forgive past mistakes, and prepare to move forward towards a healthier, more fulfilling life without regret.

Envision a future where you replace doubt with certainty, committing to make positive changes no matter the obstacles. You want to improve, and the time to begin is now. Starting from this moment, you've chosen to respect and take care of yourself. It's time to tap into your health reserves and promise never to revert to the habits that have negatively impacted your life. Look in the mirror, say it aloud, shout if you have to: NEVER AGAIN.

## A for ARBITRAGE

Life is a cascade of choices, each nudging us closer to our goals or further away. The essence lies in learning to make more thoughtful decisions, propelling us towards becoming our best selves. This notion is especially pertinent in the realm of fat loss, where arbitrage, the art of leveraging beneficial differences, can be instrumental.

One example of arbitrage is managing time and energy. For instance, waking up early or using meal prep services can free up time for healthier habits, a vital aspect of creating the calorie deficit needed for fat loss.

Arbitrage also helps balance the costs and benefits of various fat loss methods. While costly programs or supplements may be attractive, it's important to assess their value-for-money. Investing in a gym or a personal trainer, despite initial expenses, can offer greater benefits in the long run.

The concept aids in balancing immediate versus long-term gains. Although quick results may allure, sustainable lifestyle changes generally yield healthier, more enduring outcomes.

In dietary choices too, arbitrage plays a role. Healthier foods might cost more, but consciously choosing them and looking for deals on fresh produce can render long-term health dividends.

Lastly, arbitrage allows weighing the effort-versus-reward balance in fat loss. The journey is tough, necessitating commitment and discipline, but the rewards—enhanced health, boosted confidence, and a sense of accomplishment—are profound.

In a nutshell, by incorporating arbitrage into our decision-making process, we can make strategic choices leading to fat loss goals. The journey may be arduous, but the boon of improved health and wellness is priceless.

## A For AUTOLYSIS

Autolysis, derived from the Greek words meaning 'self' and 'to break down,' is a biological process where cells self-deteriorate through the release of their own enzymes. This cellular self-destruction is a crucial part of the cell life cycle, playing a pivotal role in renewing cells and maintaining overall cellular health. It ensures that older or damaged cells are replaced, facilitating new cell growth.

In a healthy state, this process is well-regulated and constructive. However, when cells are unwell or damaged, this balance can tip, leading to uncontrolled autolysis, potentially indicating disease or damage.

Autolysis also has important implications in digestion. In our small intestine, pancreatic enzymes carry out autolysis, helping to break down food for nutrient absorption. This aspect of autolysis plays a crucial role in the overall digestive process.

Medically, autolysis is useful for diagnosing various diseases or conditions. It enables the measurement of enzyme activity in cells, providing valuable insights into cellular health. It can also be induced to remove dead or damaged cells, promoting the growth of new, healthy cells.

In essence, autolysis is a complex yet fundamental process of cellular life. While a part of natural cell turnover, it can also signal cellular damage or illness. A deep understanding of autolysis is essential for a thorough grasp of cellular biology and could prove instrumental in devising treatments for diverse diseases and conditions.

## A for AUTOPHAGY

Autophagy, essentially cellular "self-eating," is a vital process that cleanses our cells by eliminating unwanted or damaged components. This helps maintain cellular balance, regulate metabolism, and handle stress.

In autophagy, a double-membrane structure, the autophagosome, envelops targeted cellular material. The autophagosome fuses with enzyme-filled organelles, and lysosomes, breaking down the captured material. The resulting components are then recycled within the cell, providing energy or raw materials for new cellular structures.

The regulation of autophagy, performed by proteins and signaling pathways, ensures its proper functioning. This process is key to maintaining cellular health and staving off diseases like cancer, neurodegenerative disorders, and metabolic conditions. Impairments in autophagy can gravely affect cell function and survival, potentially leading to severe diseases.

Autophagy can be triggered by factors such as nutrient scarcity, oxidative stress, and pathogen invasion. Certain drugs and compounds like rapamycin, known to stimulate autophagy, have been employed in treating diseases, including certain cancers and autoimmune disorders.

In essence, autophagy is crucial for cellular homeostasis and preventing disease development. Its complex regulation involving multiple steps and signaling pathways is a vibrant area of research, helping to understand its role in health and disease. Knowledge about autophagy's significance in maintaining cellular health may lead to new therapies to address a gamut of diseases affecting human health.

## A for AWARENESS

Recognizing the need for change is the first step towards becoming fit. It's crucial to understand that being overweight is often the symptom, not the root cause, of a larger problem. If you're carrying excess weight, it signifies you're consuming more calories than your body can burn, storing surplus energy as fat. This is a neutral process, like gravity; if you over consume calories consistently, weight gain is the inevitable outcome.

However, this only scratches the surface. The real challenge is to delve into the reasons behind these lifestyle choices. Understanding why you've been consuming more than necessary, why you didn't stop, and what has hindered your fat loss attempts is critical.

A successful fat loss journey requires understanding some fundamental, immutable laws of the human body. They are like the laws of physics – unchanging, regardless of your desires. When we work against these, we're destined to gain weight, leading to the all too familiar cycle of losing and regaining weight, the dreaded 'yo-yo' effect. Exceptional genes might help some, but for most of us, understanding and respecting these laws is key to sustainable fat loss.

This book aims to equip you with the necessary information to overcome these challenges. We'll explore these unchangeable laws of the body, common pitfalls, and effective strategies to address these issues. The goal is to offer a path to a healthier lifestyle, guided by knowledge and understanding. By adhering to a few simple rules, achieving long-term fitness becomes a more attainable goal.

# B

## B for BACTERIUM

We house more bacteria in our bodies than our own cells, about 38 trillion on average! While this might seem alarming, these bacteria play vital roles in our health. They inhabit everywhere, including our skin, mouth, and blood, but most importantly, our gut microbiota.

Our gut microbiota, consisting of bacteria residing in our colon, is particularly crucial. These microorganisms fortify our colon barrier, preventing harmful substances like chemicals, heavy metals, endocrine receptors (found in most processed foods), and plastic from infiltrating our system. If this barrier is compromised, these damaging substances can cause various health issues.

The specifics of these bacteria's benefits are challenging to explain, given our ongoing understanding of their interactions and functions. However, they're undeniably essential for maintaining our health and well-being.

Sadly, our human microbiome, incredibly vital, has been in severe decline over the last 40 years. This decline correlates with an increase in aging, bodily and psychological diseases, brain fog, stress, and more. This degradation is largely due to our modern lifestyle—encompassing stress, inadequate recovery, and consumption of processed foods with insufficient intake of natural foods.

Ironically, our supposed advanced lifestyle with access to an unprecedented wealth of information has become detrimental to our bodies.

The remedy, discussed in this book, is simple. It's crucial to understand bacteria's significance in our bodies, especially our gut, and the importance of not only preventing its destruction but nurturing and maintaining its health over time.

## B for BECOMING THE BEST VERSION OF YOURSELF

B&B Publishing stands for Becoming Better. This book is here to help you on your journey to becoming the best version of yourself. Our mission is to assist you in seizing every opportunity life has to offer. However, we understand that this journey must begin somewhere. That somewhere is by reclaiming your health, beauty, and resetting your mindset. Only then can you achieve excellence in every aspect of your life.

Without a functional body, excellence will always remain out of reach. You may find yourself struggling to achieve your physical, professional, or family goals. It could be that you're constantly tired, unfocused, uncomfortable, or even too lazy. These issues can become a hindrance, preventing you from reaching your full potential. That's why we present to you the ABCs of Fat Loss. It's a set of guidelines designed to help you overcome these issues and achieve your desired body and clarity of mind.

The ABCs of Fat Loss is more than just a physical transformation. It's a transformative experience that can help you take control of your life. With the right mindset, anything is possible. The protocol will give you the tools to transform your body, enabling you to achieve more than you ever thought possible. It will allow you to make healthy and informed choices that will set you on a path of personal growth and development.

We urge you to take the first step toward your journey of becoming the best version of yourself. Adopt the ABCs of Fat Loss protocol and watch as it transforms every aspect of your life. The benefits go beyond just physical transformation. The protocol can help you gain mental clarity and develop a positive mindset, leading to increased productivity and success in your personal and professional life.

We understand that embarking on this journey can be daunting. However, we encourage you to embrace the process, knowing that the end result is a better you. Take control of your life, and start working toward your goals today. The B&B edition is here to guide you every step of the way, so take the first step and get ready to become the best version of yourself.

## B for BEHAVIOR

Our diet has a powerful impact on our overall well-being—physically and psychologically. Our food choices can significantly influence our mood, work performance, and even earnings. Moving towards a diet that emphasizes natural foods, with less salt, sugar, and processed items, can enhance our health and quickly lift our mood. Studies suggest that proper nutrition can significantly lessen symptoms of mental health issues like depression, ADHD, anxiety, and bipolar disorder, with some individuals even achieving complete remission through a diet rich in fresh, plant-based foods.

Moreover, dietary habits can also shape life outcomes. For instance, consuming high-sugar foods can lead to blood sugar spikes, inciting anger and aggression. Unhealthy eating and sedentary lifestyles can have serious ramifications, with links to conditions like ADHD, Alzheimer's, diabetes, Parkinson's, and depression.

Yet, hope exists. In a study, prisoners who adopted healthier diets showed notable improvements in mental and physical health, and their likelihood to re-offend was reduced after release. Eating healthily not only prevents diseases but also improves mood, cognitive function, and overall life quality.

In conclusion, adopting healthier dietary habits is pivotal for enhancing mental and physical health. The journey starts by gaining a deeper understanding of nutrition and beneficial foods. Remember, the objective isn't just to avoid the negatives but to nurture the best version of yourself and lead a fulfilling life.

## B for BELIEVE

Numerous studies have demonstrated the intimate connection between the body and the mind. It's clear that the way we think can have a profound impact on how our bodies react. Our thoughts and emotions can trigger the release of hormones such as adrenaline and dopamine that can help us achieve our goals. It's important to note, however, that setting realistic goals is crucial to avoid disappointment and feelings of failure.

The key is to have faith in oneself and commit to the process, no matter how long it may take or how difficult it may seem. This means believing that you can achieve the body and lifestyle that you desire and being willing to put in the work and make the necessary changes to get there.

It's crucial to break free from unhealthy habits and make positive changes that will benefit both your physical and mental well-being. This might mean making changes to your diet, increasing your exercise routine, or taking steps to reduce stress and anxiety in your life. It's important to keep in mind that small, incremental changes can have a big impact over time, and it's never too late to start.

Ultimately, the goal should be to reach a state of balance and harmony between the mind and body, allowing for optimal health and well-being. With patience, dedication, and a positive attitude, it's possible to overcome even the most stubborn of obstacles and achieve the body and lifestyle that you deserve. So, believe in yourself, commit to the process, and watch as you become the best version of yourself that you can be.

## B for BENEFITS

Maintaining good health and specifically following the ABCs of Fat Loss can bring a multitude of benefits. Firstly, life expectancy can be significantly extended. A health-conscious individual can potentially live decades longer than one who neglects their well-being, providing more time with loved ones, opportunities for exploration, and the potential to create a greater impact.

Secondly, nurturing health boosts daily energy levels. Losing extra weight and eating balanced meals can provide you with the vitality needed to engage in your passions and accomplish meaningful goals.

The third benefit is the elimination of fatigue. Prioritizing health allows you to start each day refreshed and energized, ready to face the day's hurdles.

Fourthly, improving diet and physical condition can alleviate various physical ailments such as aches, breathing issues, and more severe health problems like diabetes and high blood pressure. It also helps combat psychological issues like depression and brain fog, leading to clearer thinking and a more positive outlook.

Lastly, taking care of yourself can positively impact your finances in two ways. Firstly, you can save on medical bills and junk food costs, leading to potential investments for your future financial health. Secondly, physical fitness can open doors for career advancement and expand your social and professional circles.

In conclusion, adopting a healthier lifestyle offers numerous benefits: extended lifespan, increased energy, reduced fatigue, improved physical and mental well-being, and financial advantages. Start investing in your health today to reap these rewards and lead a more fulfilling life.

## B for BINGE EATING

Binge eating involves excessively consuming food in a short span, often leading to adverse effects on one's health, self-esteem, and even finances. This behavior stems from both physical and psychological triggers.

Physically, binge eating often arises from a drop in blood sugar levels. Consuming high-sugar foods prompts an insulin surge, which then leads to a sharp drop in blood sugar, signaling your brain to eat more. Your brain typically craves fast-energy foods like fries or chocolate, which further exacerbates the blood sugar fluctuation cycle. This reaction can lead you to eat excessively and frequently, significantly surpassing your daily calorie intake.

Psychologically, binge eating can offer temporary comfort. Junk foods stimulate dopamine production in our brains, providing immediate gratification. However, this pleasure is short-lived and can lead to addictive patterns.

To curb binge eating, first, practice mindfulness. When you feel a binge episode coming, pause, take deep breaths, and reflect on your stress levels. Understanding the process your body is undergoing can help you respond to it better. Ask yourself if you're genuinely hungry, why you feel that way, and what consequences may arise from indulging in unhealthy eating. Rationalize your situation and remind yourself of your health goals.

If these steps aren't enough, drinking a large glass of water and waiting a bit can help curb the urge. If hunger persists, opt for a healthy snack, such as vegetables or a non-sugary source of fats. By understanding and implementing these strategies, you can break the binge-eating cycle and maintain healthier eating habits.

## B for BLOOD

Blood, the body's lifeline, performs critical functions like transporting nutrients, removing waste, and linking all organs and systems. Analyzing it offers valuable insights into an individual's health and lifestyle. Blood tests can detect vitamin and nutrient deficiencies, which might cause fatigue or obstruct personal goals. They can also spot potential liver issues, a primary cause of death worldwide, and estimate heart attack risk via D-dimer levels. Hence, regular blood analysis is crucial for maintaining health and tracking wellness.

For those starting the ABCs of Fat Loss protocol, a blood test is highly recommended. It serves as a safety check, evaluating your overall health before initiating new regimes. It can also act as a wake-up call, emphasizing the urgent need for self-care and breaking unhealthy habits. Furthermore, blood tests enable effective progress tracking, letting you measure health improvement efforts over time.

Maintaining blood health is key to overall wellness. Your blood reflects your lifestyle, decisions, and habits. A balanced diet, sufficient hydration, regular exercise, and abstaining from harmful habits like smoking and excessive alcohol intake significantly enhance blood health.

In conclusion, blood plays an indispensable role in body function, and blood analysis is a vital health tool. It provides crucial insights about our health, spotlighting areas needing attention. Prioritizing blood health and making lifestyle choices that promote a healthy body is of utmost importance.

## B for BLOOD ANALYSIS

Blood analysis is a crucial element in the fat loss journey, often overlooked in favor of traditional diet and exercise. It delves deeper into metabolic functioning, hormonal balance, and nutrient deficiencies, often the hidden culprits of unsuccessful fat loss. Insulin, which regulates blood sugar, plays a key role in fat loss. Excessive carbohydrates or insulin resistance can boost insulin levels, causing weight gain, which fasting insulin tests can detect, helping guide dietary changes. Similarly, cortisol, the stress hormone, can affect metabolism and energy balance, potentially leading to weight gain. Tests can reveal if stress is impeding fat loss and suggest stress-reducing solutions. Nutrient deficiencies, such as vitamin D or iron, can also affect fat loss. Tests can identify these deficiencies, leading to advice on increasing intake. Blood analysis is thus an essential tool for a comprehensive understanding of health issues that impede fat loss and allows for targeted strategy formulation. If you're struggling with fat loss, a blood test might be the key to uncover and tackle underlying issues.

## B for BLOOD CIRCULATION

Healthy blood circulation is a cornerstone of fat loss and overall health. Accumulated body fat can hinder blood flow, leading to health complications. However, fat loss can improve circulation, reducing pressure on the heart and expanding blood vessels. This promotes better function and efficiency of muscles, organs, and tissues. Regular exercise bolsters circulation by enhancing blood flow and vessel quantity, which supports fat-burning and muscle development. Lifestyle alterations, like smoking cessation, alcohol moderation, and stress control, also affect blood circulation, improving or inhibiting it. Nutrition is vital as well - a diet rich in nutrients but low in processed foods and saturated fats boosts circulation efficiency and minimizes heart disease risk. Despite these benefits, rapid fat loss can lead to reduced blood sugar levels, causing dizziness or lightheadedness. Hence, a gradual, supervised approach is advised. To summarize, fat loss, exercise, stress management, and a balanced diet contribute to better circulation and lower cardiovascular risk. Yet, always seek professional guidance for safe and effective fat loss.

## B for BLOOD PRESSURE

Blood pressure, indicating the force against artery walls, is a critical health measure. Ideal readings are typically below 120/80 mmHg, while consistent higher readings, or hypertension, can lead to severe health issues like heart disease and stroke. Hypertension, often symptomless and called the "silent killer," is a leading cause of death globally. Risk factors include being overweight, inactivity, smoking, alcohol abuse, and an unhealthy diet. Managing hypertension largely involves lifestyle modifications like maintaining a healthy weight, regular exercise, quitting smoking, reducing alcohol, and following a nutritious diet low in sodium. Medication might be required, with choices varying based on hypertension severity and other health conditions. Regular blood pressure monitoring is crucial for early detection, and annual or more frequent checks are recommended. Symptoms like headaches or shortness of breath warrant immediate medical attention. In conclusion, maintaining healthy blood pressure through lifestyle changes, medication, and regular checks is vital, with prevention primarily focusing on leading a healthy lifestyle.

## B for BODY MEMORY

Body memory, the capacity of our bodies to remember past experiences, significantly influences fat loss and weight maintenance. It affects our eating and exercise patterns, stress responses, and sleep habits. By making conscious decisions, we can modify these patterns. If we habitually consume high-calorie, fatty foods, our body memory triggers cravings for these, even during fat loss. By slowly reducing portions and choosing nutrient-dense foods, we can retrain our bodies towards healthier preferences. Gradually incorporating exercise into a sedentary lifestyle can similarly reprogram body memory to appreciate physical activity. Stress influences body memory by prompting hormone releases that stimulate appetite, often leading to overeating. Practices like meditation can teach our bodies healthier stress responses, helping to curb unhealthy food cravings. Sleep deprivation similarly affects body memory by triggering hunger-inducing hormones, emphasizing the need for good sleep patterns. In conclusion, understanding and altering body memory through healthier food choices, regular exercise, stress management, and ample sleep can promote sustainable fat loss. It's a gradual process requiring patience, but the rewards are long-term health and weight control.

## B for BRAINS

New findings suggest we possess three "brains" in our bodies - one each in our head, heart, and stomach, revolutionizing our understanding of the human body. This fascinating discovery reveals neurons exist not just in our brains but also in our hearts and stomachs.

This means our physical and psychological conditions result not only from our thoughts but also from our diet and emotions. The so-called heart and gut brains, defined by the neurons in these organs, have a significant impact on our overall health, being greatly influenced by our dietary choices and physical activity levels.

Essentially, maintaining a balanced diet, positive thoughts, and regular physical activity is paramount for our well-being. Consuming foods rich in fiber, vitamins, and minerals, which are good for the gut, is vital. Equally important is regular exercise, like brisk walking or cycling, beneficial for heart health, and choosing enjoyable activities ensures consistency.

Our mindset also significantly affects our health. Negative thoughts can trigger stress and anxiety, leading to numerous physical and mental health issues. Conversely, positivity can reduce stress, enhancing our overall health.

In summary, the discovery of our hearts and gut brains expands our comprehension of human physiology. It emphasizes the necessity of mindful eating, positive thinking, and regular physical activity for holistic health. By adopting positive changes in diet, lifestyle, and thought patterns, we optimize our potential for a fulfilling life.

## B for BREAKEVEN

Starting a new diet can be tough, especially in the first few days when cravings are at their peak and energy may be low. However, it's vital to endure these initial difficulties, as the rewards of a healthy diet are tremendous. With persistence, you'll experience notable changes: cravings will diminish, you'll feel more in control of your food choices, and as your body adapts, energy levels will rise, bringing greater alertness and focus. A healthier lifestyle might seem daunting initially, but with time, it will become more manageable and natural. By adhering to your diet plan, you'll reap benefits such as fat loss, mood enhancement, and increased energy. The key to success lies in understanding past struggles with maintaining a healthy diet. This book will offer insights into potential obstacles that may have led to past dietary failures. Armed with this knowledge, you'll be better prepared to make positive changes and maintain your diet. Remember, significant lifestyle changes can be tough, and it's essential to be patient with yourself. The concepts in this book may take time to fully grasp, but with perseverance, you'll be on the path to achieving your goals. In conclusion, while the first diet days can be challenging, pushing through brings remarkable benefits. This book will provide the necessary knowledge and understanding to help you break old habits and embrace a healthier lifestyle for lasting success.

## B for BREAKING THE CYCLE BEFORE IT'S TOO LATE

Embarking on a fat loss journey can sometimes result in unhealthy eating patterns and overeating, which can be detrimental to physical and mental health. Recognizing and addressing these habits before they escalate is crucial. This requires self-awareness and honesty, alongside creating healthier eating routines. Regular, balanced meals help keep blood sugar levels stable and prevent extreme hunger that may trigger overeating. Being aware of and managing physical and emotional symptoms tied to overeating, such as stomach pain or fatigue, can prevent further harm and promote a healthier relationship with food. Mindfulness about what you eat and portion sizes is key. Prioritizing whole foods over processed ones and practicing portion control can ward off health issues related to overeating. Don't hesitate to seek professional help if needed. A dietitian, healthcare provider, or therapist can provide valuable support, helping manage emotions, stress, and creating a balanced eating plan. In summary, successful fat loss requires breaking harmful eating cycles, adopting healthier habits, recognizing physical and emotional triggers, making mindful food choices, and accessing professional support when necessary. It's a journey requiring patience, self-compassion, and a learning mindset.

## B for BUTTERFLY EFFECT

The Butterfly Effect – the notion that small changes can lead to substantial outcomes – holds significant relevance to fat loss. It emphasizes that each decision, regardless of scale, has an impact on your fat loss progression. For example, opting for a salad instead of a burger might seem inconsequential, yet it affects your overall calorie count and promotes fat loss.

The Butterfly Effect also highlights the interconnectedness of life aspects; your diet choices affect your energy levels and, subsequently, your ability to exercise and make future healthier decisions.

However, it can also work adversely; small unhealthy choices, such as regular high-calorie snacking, can accumulate and hamper fat loss.

Harnessing the Butterfly Effect favorably involves creating healthy habits – consistent small positive choices leading to a routine of beneficial behaviors, like meal prepping, choosing healthy snacks, staying hydrated, and exercising regularly.

It's also crucial to approach the Butterfly Effect with self-compassion. Occasional lapses are natural and shouldn't deter you; recognizing them and bouncing back maintains progress.

Lastly, our choices can also influence others, creating a beneficial ripple effect that encourages healthier practices in our community.

To sum up, the Butterfly Effect significantly affects our fat loss journey. Embracing its power through daily small positive choices, and self-compassion can foster our progress, help achieve fat loss goals, and promote a healthier lifestyle for ourselves and our community.

# C

## C for CAFFEINE

Caffeine is a common element in many diets, but excessive intake can negatively impact fat loss efforts. Although moderate caffeine can increase calorie burn due to heightened heart rate, blood pressure, and stress hormone production, it can also impair insulin sensitivity, complicating blood sugar regulation.

Contrary to popular belief, caffeine doesn't always suppress appetite. Some individuals may feel hungrier after caffeine intake, leading to overeating. Moreover, caffeinated beverages often contain high levels of calories and sugar, promoting weight gain.

Sleep disruption, another concern with caffeine, affects hunger and satiety hormones. Insufficient sleep can spur overeating and escalate stress levels, contributing to weight gain.

Caffeine can also cause digestive issues and dehydration, making it hard to stick to a healthy diet.

While caffeine might offer some benefits like increased energy and calorie burning, the possible negative impacts often outweigh these gains. Particularly for those sensitive to caffeine or with existing health conditions, limiting or avoiding caffeine is recommended.

Favorable alternatives to caffeine include nutrient-rich foods, sufficient hydration, regular exercise, and adequate sleep.

To sum up, while moderate caffeine is generally safe, excessive intake can impede fat loss. It impacts metabolism, appetite, sleep, and digestion, potentially leading to weight gain. Focusing on healthier habits and alternatives can bolster fat loss efforts and support a healthy weight.

## C for CALORIE & CONVERSION

Calories, a measure of energy in food and drinks and our physical activity, are crucial for understanding nutrition and managing weight. Essential for body function, calories, when consumed in excess, lead to weight gain, with surplus energy stored as fat. Conversely, a calorie deficit, achieved by burning more calories than consumed, can result in fat loss.

Understanding basal metabolic rate (BMR) - the energy needed for basic body functions - can help comprehend calorie needs. Factors like age, gender, height, weight, and activity level affect BMR, which helps calculate total daily energy expenditure (TDEE). A calorie deficit requires consuming fewer calories than our TDEE.

Notably, calorie quality matters. Nutrient-rich foods like fruits, vegetables, lean proteins, and whole grains offer essential vitamins, minerals, and fiber with relatively fewer calories. Conversely, foods high in added sugars, unhealthy fats, and refined carbs are often calorie-dense but nutritionally poor. Limiting these "empty calorie" foods is essential for a healthy diet.

Understanding how physical activity burns calories can also help. Different activities burn varying calorie amounts, with factors like weight, pace, and intensity influencing calorie burn. While strength training and yoga might not burn as many calories as cardiovascular exercises, they provide unique health benefits like muscle building and flexibility improvement.

In short, understanding and managing calories is key to successful nutrition and weight management. Achieving a calorie deficit, opting for nutrient-dense foods, and regular physical activity all contribute to healthier living and fat loss success.

## C for CATABOLISM

Catabolism is a metabolic process that breaks down complex molecules into smaller units, releasing energy for cellular use. This process is crucial for energy metabolism and life maintenance. It's a counter-process to anabolism, which builds larger molecules from smaller ones.

In catabolism, enzymes break down large molecules like carbohydrates into glucose, lipids into fatty acids and glycerol, and proteins into amino acids. These components are further degraded and oxidized, producing ATP, the cell's primary energy source.

Various hormones and enzymes regulate catabolic pathways, ensuring controlled and adaptable energy production to meet the cell's needs. For instance, glucagon triggers the breakdown of glycogen in the liver, while insulin promotes glucose storage as glycogen in the liver and muscles.

Catabolism also aids in recycling cellular components, as unnecessary or damaged proteins are broken down into amino acids, which can be repurposed to create new proteins. Moreover, some small molecules produced by catabolism serve as building blocks for biosynthesis pathways, enabling the construction of larger molecules.

In conclusion, catabolism is an integral part of metabolism. It helps cells generate energy, recycle components, and synthesize new molecules. Disruptions in catabolic pathways can lead to metabolic disorders like diabetes, obesity, and some types of cancer.

## C For CELL

The human body is a complex system of trillions of cells each performing vital functions. One key player in fat loss is the mitochondria, the cellular components responsible for energy production. They transform nutrients and oxygen into ATP, the primary energy source. Cells with higher energy requirements, like muscle and brown fat cells, contain more mitochondria.

Boosting mitochondrial count via regular aerobic exercise can enhance calorie burning, aiding in fat loss.

Insulin resistance is another crucial element in fat loss. Insulin maintains blood sugar levels by prompting cells to absorb glucose for energy or storage. However, insulin resistance, prevalent in overweight or obese people, disrupts this process, leading to elevated blood sugar levels. Maintaining a healthy weight, limiting carbohydrate and sugar intake, and exercising regularly can improve insulin sensitivity.

Chronic inflammation is also linked to obesity and can obstruct fat loss efforts. It disrupts appetite regulation and metabolism. To mitigate inflammation, opt for an anti-inflammatory diet rich in fruits, vegetables, whole grains, lean proteins, and Omega-3 fatty acids found in fatty fish, flaxseed, and chia seeds. Regular exercise also reduces inflammation by controlling cytokine production.

In essence, understanding the role of mitochondria, insulin resistance, and inflammation in cellular function is critical for effective fat loss. Incorporating strategies to increase mitochondrial activity, improve insulin sensitivity, and reduce inflammation through diet and exercise can provide a holistic approach to fat loss and overall health.

## C for CHANGES

Embarking on the journey to achieve your goals necessitates lifestyle changes, both minor and major. If you want different results, you can't stick to the same routines; change is essential. But what does it truly mean to change, and how should you go about it?

To understand change, think of life as a journey along a path. To change is to shift your direction from a losing path to a winning one, requiring energy to drive this movement. The necessary changes could include adjusting your diet, replacing harmful hobbies, or modifying your workout routine.

Before you alter your course, you need to evaluate your current position, your desired destination, and the route you wish to follow. Is it the quickest, safest, or most enjoyable route?

The quickest path is often the most challenging, dangerous, and has the lowest success rate. It's akin to crash diets, which often result in fatigue and disappointment. The safest path, while taking a bit longer, assures you'll reach your destination without the risk of having to backtrack.

The most enjoyable path might not get you to your goal as quickly but offers a fun and memorable journey. For instance, Pilates or Zumba might be less effective than High-Intensity Interval Training (HIIT) in terms of calorie burning or muscle building, but they're more enjoyable.

Ultimately, the choice of the path and pace lies with you. My role is to provide information on each path, enabling you to make informed decisions. The key is to make healthier choices than the previous day and to keep moving forward. Don't worry, all necessary information will be provided in due time.

## C for CHOICES

Our life's outcomes largely depend on the choices we make. Bad choices can lead to damaging effects such as broken relationships, financial issues, and legal troubles, also taking a toll on our mental health. People often make poor choices due to a lack of awareness about the potential repercussions or succumbing to peer pressure. Impulsiveness and short-term gratification also play a role.

Bad choices can result in severe, lasting consequences such as legal penalties, financial hardship, strained relationships, or even irreversible outcomes like accidents. Those battling addiction or mental health problems may also be more susceptible to making poor decisions.

Just as with life in general, our choices significantly affect our health. Consuming processed foods, smoking, heavy drinking, and disregarding safety precautions can contribute to obesity, diabetes, heart disease, cancer, and mental health issues.

However, the brighter side is that it's never too late to change. Developing good decision-making skills and taking positive steps can drastically transform our lives. This applies to our health as well. By adopting healthier habits like a balanced diet, regular exercise, quitting smoking, and reducing alcohol, we can boost our physical and mental health. It's also vital to seek professional help when dealing with mental health issues or addiction.

In a nutshell, while bad choices can lead to dire consequences, positive change is always within reach. By making better decisions, we can enhance our health, well-being, and mitigate the risk of chronic diseases.

## C FOR CLARITY

Bravo on embarking on your health journey! This isn't just a quick-fix diet, it's a lifelong commitment to wellness. Before, lack of a clear roadmap might have led to dead-ends. Now, with a defined path, specific goals, and practical strategies, you're ready for success. Prioritize health, embrace the process, and remember, this is a lasting lifestyle transformation.

Swapping old habits for new ones is key—cook fresh meals, prioritize rest, engage in regular physical activity, and replace destructive behaviors with healthy alternatives. You're shifting towards a life that focuses on lasting wellness rather than short-lived pleasure.

Every decision should resonate with your ultimate goal. Avoid falling into the trap of momentary indulgences and concentrate on the bigger picture. It's not about deprivation, it's about abundance; choosing nutritious options that feed your body and soul rather than temporary, unhealthy pleasures.

Your journey to successful fat loss and health restoration hinges on two elements—clarity and alignment. Clarity involves a well-defined plan, timelines, and strategies, while alignment ensures your decisions align with your long-term goals. Move away from the mentality of scarcity and step into a mindset of abundance, making nourishing choices that bring life and vitality. This book is your companion on this journey, providing a step-by-step guide towards achieving your health goals and living a revitalized life.

## C for CLEANSE

Today's lifestyle, often distanced from nature, burdens our bodies with toxins. These interfere with our organs' function and self-cleansing abilities. Over time, toxins amass, regardless of how healthy we live. Our bodies can eliminate them, but our bustling lifestyles often deprive them of the required energy and time. Overweight or obese individuals may find it even harder to detoxify.

One pressing concern is fecal matter buildup in our intestines, sometimes weighing up to 50 pounds. Processed food consumption and fiber-poor diets are to blame, making digestion difficult. Excessive fecal matter can result in dangerous intestinal blockages, requiring surgery. In severe cases, it can even affect breathing and speaking.

Additionally, having excessive fecal matter can lead to stretch marks, skin issues, knee and back problems, breathing difficulties, and psychological conditions. This buildup can limit the brain's nutrient and oxygen supply, leading to depression and burnout. Fecal matter toxins can infiltrate the bloodstream, leading to diverse health problems, including cancer.

Counteracting these issues requires concerted efforts. Prioritize eliminating processed foods, which contribute to toxin buildup. Embrace fasting, natural fiber-rich foods, and vegetable juice therapy to cleanse the intestines. Standing more often and exercising stimulates intestinal movement, aiding in waste expulsion. Hydrating adequately and considering a detox tea or herbal cleanse can further aid waste and toxin removal.

Cleansing your body and removing toxins can trigger rejuvenation and a series of positive effects. Without toxins, your body can heal and operate more efficiently. Your posture can improve, knee and back pain can diminish, your diaphragm can work better, and oxygen supply to organs can increase, boosting your energy levels and motivation. Hence, addressing toxins and fecal matter buildup is vital for overall health and well-being. Adopting various solutions will empower your body's natural detoxification process, leading to a healthier, rejuvenated self.

You will be able to find everything you need through the following website:

https://www.the10sprotocol.com/detox

## C for COLD BENEFICE

There's a growing fascination with using cold exposure for fat loss, a method involving subjecting the body to low temperatures via cold showers, ice baths, or spending time in cold rooms. It may sound daunting, but research indicates it could be beneficial for shedding weight.

Cold exposure may boost the body's metabolic rate as the body strives to maintain its core temperature, thus burning more calories and potentially aiding in fat loss. It can also activate brown fat, known for burning calories rather than storing them, thereby further promoting fat loss.

Another merit of cold exposure is its potential to reduce inflammation. Chronic inflammation has been linked to several health issues, including obesity, and cold temperatures may help decrease these inflammatory markers in the body.

In terms of mental benefits, cold exposure can foster mental resilience and discipline, positively influencing diet and exercise habits. The accomplishment of enduring discomfort can also serve as a powerful motivator.

However, cold exposure isn't a standalone solution for fat loss. It should complement a healthy diet and regular exercise. Those with specific health conditions should consult a doctor before beginning cold exposure.

Implementing cold exposure into a fat loss routine can be done by gradually reducing shower or bath water temperature. More intense methods include time in a cryotherapy chamber or ice bath, which could provide more significant benefits.

In conclusion, cold exposure, when combined with other healthy habits, can be a useful tool in a fat loss routine. It can enhance the metabolic rate, activate brown fat, reduce inflammation, and build mental strength. However, it should be used responsibly, with individuals with underlying health conditions consulting professionals before starting.

COLD SHOWER

Cold showers can assist fat loss by increasing the body's metabolic rate. When the body is exposed to cold, it strives to maintain its core temperature, which can enhance calorie burn and potentially contribute to fat loss. Cold showers might also activate brown fat, a type of fat that burns calories instead of storing them.

Cold showers might also help reduce inflammation. Chronic inflammation is often linked to health problems, including obesity. Cold temperatures have been shown to lower inflammatory markers, potentially aiding fat loss.

Aside from physiological benefits, cold showers can also foster mental resilience and discipline. Enduring the discomfort of cold showers can impact other areas, such as diet and exercise habits. The sense of achievement from managing the discomfort can act as a powerful motivator.

However, cold showers aren't a panacea for fat loss and should be part of a healthy diet and exercise routine. Those with certain health conditions, like Raynaud's disease or diabetes, should seek medical advice before incorporating cold showers.

Implementing cold showers in a fat loss routine can be gradual, starting with lukewarm water and gradually making it colder. Another method is alternating hot and cold water during a shower, ending with a cold rinse to improve circulation and reduce inflammation.

Adjusting to cold showers may initially be challenging but, with consistent practice, the discomfort can become more bearable.

In conclusion, cold showers can be an effective tool in fat loss, increasing metabolic rate, activating brown fat, reducing inflammation, and building mental strength. Coupled with other healthy habits, they can support sustainable fat loss. Those with specific health conditions should consult their doctor before attempting. Despite the initial discomfort, incorporating cold showers into your routine can be a powerful step towards achieving your fat loss goals.

ICE BATH

Ice baths may be an effective tool for enhancing fat loss by boosting metabolism. As the body strives to maintain its core temperature in cold conditions, it burns more calories, which can expedite fat loss. Ice baths can also reduce inflammation, a natural response linked to numerous health issues, including obesity. By lessening inflammation, ice baths might contribute to fat loss and better overall health.

Interestingly, ice baths can activate brown fat, which burns calories rather than storing them, further aiding fat loss. Cold exposure has been proven to stimulate brown fat activity, making ice baths a viable fat loss strategy.

Beyond physical benefits, ice baths can foster mental resilience. The initial discomfort of plunging into icy water can bolster mental fortitude, influencing other areas like diet and exercise habits. The sense of achievement from enduring an ice bath can also be a strong motivator for fat loss.

Incorporating ice baths into a fat loss routine can be gradual, starting with lukewarm water and progressively making it colder. Another method involves alternating between hot and cold water during a bath, ending with a cold rinse, which may improve circulation and reduce inflammation.

Ice baths can initially be uncomfortable, but consistent practice can make the sensation more manageable over time. Caution is advised, particularly for those with health conditions like Raynaud's disease or diabetes. Consult a doctor before starting ice baths, and avoid prolonged exposure to cold temperatures.

In summary, ice baths can be a valuable component of a fat loss routine, increasing metabolism, activating brown fat, reducing inflammation, and promoting mental resilience. When used responsibly and alongside other healthy habits, they can help attain fat loss goals sustainably. Those with certain health conditions should consult their doctor before starting. If you're game for a challenge, consider adding ice baths to your routine - take the plunge and witness the benefits unfold!

You will be able to find everything you need through the following website:

https://bit.ly/THE10SCOLDBATH

https://www.the10sprotocol.com/sport

## C for COMFORT ZONE

**"The comfort zone is the place where all your dreams go to die"**

Overcoming the comfort zone is pivotal for effective fat loss. The comfort zone, a psychological space marked by safety and predictability, becomes a significant roadblock in our fat loss journey. Its allure lies in familiarity and ease, where routines and habits go unquestioned and unchanged. However, staying in this zone impedes progress, maintaining the status quo rather than fostering growth and improvement.

Escaping the comfort zone entails embracing discomfort. Trying new foods, exercises, and routines is crucial. This leap into the unfamiliar may be daunting but can also ignite excitement and discovery. It propels us into uncharted territory, opening up a world of novel experiences and self-understanding.

The comfort zone is tough to leave because it offers familiarity. We can predict outcomes and handle challenges adeptly. However, stepping into the unknown is not just disconcerting, but also an opportunity to learn and grow. We must be open to new approaches and experiences, even if they intimidate us initially.

Moreover, the comfort zone shields us from facing our fears and weaknesses. To break out, we must confront them head-on, however uncomfortable it might be. This confrontation paves the way for growth and overcoming limitations.

Busting out of the comfort zone means we need to acknowledge our fears, address our weaknesses, and learn from our mistakes. Accepting feedback and criticism is also key. Although challenging, this leads to personal growth and self-improvement.

In summary, while the comfort zone may offer safety and control, it deters fat loss efforts. To break out, we must challenge ourselves, be open to unfamiliar experiences, and confront our fears head-on. It provides an avenue for personal growth, enabling us to reach the best version of ourselves. So, step out of your comfort zone, embrace the unknown, and remember you're equipped to win. Strike "giving up" from your vocabulary and surround yourself with positivity and support.

## C for COMPLIMENTS

Starting the ABCs of Fat Loss Protocol can result in rapid transformations, especially for those with substantial excess weight. It's not uncommon to shed several pounds in the initial weeks, coupled with noticeable improvements like better skin complexion, enhanced eye brightness, fresher breath, and improved posture. Your energy levels might skyrocket and your mental clarity sharpen. While you may spot these changes early, others might take a little longer to notice your transformation.

Remember, everyone's journey to fat loss is unique and progress visible to others may vary. Typically, people who see you often might start noticing significant changes in your appearance around 6-8 weeks into the program. By this time, you could have already lost a substantial amount of weight, around 20-40 pounds, becoming noticeable to your close circle. People who see you less frequently might take longer, about two to three months, to observe changes, including shifts in your attitude, posture, and clothing. You may even need a wardrobe overhaul as your old clothes become too big.

Receiving compliments can act as a potent motivator, boosting your drive towards your health goals. While your focus remains on health and wellness, acknowledging recognition from others for your hard work can be invigorating. Positive feedback can serve as a tangible reminder of your progress, fueling your determination to stay committed to your fitness goals.

As you evolve on your journey, you may inspire others and become a source of guidance. Sharing your transformation story and experiences can be gratifying, potentially inspiring some to explore health and fitness careers.

In conclusion, the ABCs of Fat Loss Protocol can catalyze your transformation towards a healthier and more confident you.

Although others might take a while to notice your progress, you'll experience positive shifts in your body and mind from the get-go.

## C for COMPOUND EFFECT

The compound effect is a pivotal concept in the ABCs of Fat Loss Protocol. Its two key components, the snowball and the virtuous effects, play essential roles in health transformation.

The snowball effect, like a rolling snowball growing in size, implies that a small initial action can trigger a cascade of larger effects. This concept applies to your health journey too - whether it's the ABCs of Fat Loss Protocol, diet, or exercise. Any small initial step can spark a process that, over time, becomes formidable and impactful. Identifying what hinders you from starting or continuing your journey will be discussed later in this book, but remember, the snowball effect's power lies in taking that first step.

The virtuous effect, another essential component, is a positive feedback loop that grows over time. Consider exercise as an example. Your first workout may last only five minutes, but as you persist, your stamina increases. The initial five-minute workout that once felt tough would feel much easier compared to a one-hour workout six months later. This progressive improvement illustrates the virtuous effect.

So, as you embark on the ABCs of Fat Loss Protocol, remember that persistence is key. Acknowledge that the toughest step, deciding to start your journey, has already been taken. Keep faith in the process and continue striving, for the compound effect is at play, making each effort more potent over time.

## C for CONFRONTING YOUR PAST

Addressing fat loss requires not just a physical transformation, but also tackling the emotional and psychological factors that contribute to weight gain. A critical part of this journey is confronting your past. This process involves an honest reflection on past events and experiences that have shaped you, even the painful ones, acknowledging the negative beliefs and behaviors that could be impeding your fat loss goals.

In many cases, this confrontation means dealing with past traumas or negative experiences that might have led to unhealthy coping mechanisms, such as overeating. Acknowledging these experiences is the first step towards healing and making progress. Additionally, taking responsibility for past choices, even when difficult, is empowering, leading to a realization that you can change your life.

An important aspect of confronting your past is learning to forgive - yourself and others. Letting go of anger, guilt, and resentment helps to focus on the present and future, instead of getting stuck in the past.

Remember, confronting the past is an ongoing process demanding constant self-awareness and reflection. As you embark on your fat loss journey, you might uncover new emotions and beliefs that require attention. Be patient and gentle with yourself during this journey.

Consider seeking help from therapists or counselors, as they provide a safe space to explore emotions and process past trauma. They can also assist in developing healthy coping mechanisms. There are other resources too, like support groups, self-help books, and online communities.

In conclusion, confronting your past is vital for lasting fat loss. By addressing the psychological and emotional factors associated with weight gain, healing can begin, and progress can be achieved. It's a challenging journey, but with dedication, patience, and the right support, you can face your past and create a healthier future.

## C for COST OF OPPORTUNITY

Opportunity cost is a crucial principle in understanding the fat loss journey. It refers to the benefits we forfeit and the costs we incur by choosing a specific path. When we neglect our health, we miss out on opportunities to live a healthier, longer life, to feel confident and comfortable in our bodies, and to participate in a broader range of physical activities.

Financial expenses tied to fat loss—like gym memberships, personal training, and healthier food—are intimidating to some, yet it's vital to consider the long-term health benefits that outweigh these immediate costs. Ignoring excessive weight can lead to expensive medical treatments for obesity-related conditions.

Time and effort form another significant aspect of opportunity cost in fat loss. The process requires major lifestyle shifts—regular exercise, nutritious meals, and self-care. These changes might mean less socializing or reduced time for hobbies, but improved health and well-being are worthwhile trade-offs.

The cost of not pursuing fat loss goals is equally critical. The potential worsening of health conditions—like high blood pressure, diabetes, or heart disease—impacts the quality of life and lifespan. The opportunity for personal growth and self-improvement can also be limited.

In essence, understanding the opportunity cost in fat loss involves weighing the costs and benefits of pursuing these goals. While there are financial, time, and effort considerations, the rewards of improved health and personal growth are significant. Prioritizing long-term well-being and recognizing the value of investing in oneself is essential.

## C for CYCLE

The crux of the disparity between a fit and an unhealthy individual lies in "the cycle" – a daily routine adhered to by healthy people that maintains their fitness and energy levels. Even though they occasionally break from routine for leisure or treats, they can successfully revert to it.

They adhere to a regular workout schedule with assigned days for different activities like cardio, yoga, and weightlifting. They manage their calorie intake, ensuring a balanced consumption of proteins, lipids, and carbohydrates. Regular checks on their calendar help them stick to their gym schedules, and advanced meal planning assists in achieving nutritional goals and avoiding unhealthy snacks.

Healthy people also understand the art of indulgence. They partake in cheat meals or days without overconsumption, balancing indulgence by reverting to their routine and incorporating physical activity. This maintains their lifestyle balance without resorting to punishing diets.

Creating such a cycle is achievable. It involves consistently performing beneficial actions until they become routine. A successful day can be repeated to form a successful week, after which some measured fun is acceptable. The key is to always return to the cycle to maintain balance and achieve health and fitness goals.

# D

## D for DANGEROUSNESS

The term "diet product" often suggests a simple, fast route to fat loss, but that's a fallacy. Many of these products are, in fact, potentially harmful to health due to their synthetic ingredients, stimulants, and laxatives. Take ephedra, for example, a common ingredient found in diet products. While it's banned in the US due to adverse side effects like high blood pressure, heart palpitations, and even heart attacks, it's available elsewhere and online. Sibutramine, another ingredient, was once a weight-loss drug but got banned due to its risk of inducing heart attacks and strokes.

The use of laxatives for fat loss can also lead to dehydration, electrolyte imbalances, and colon damage over time. Unvetted synthetic ingredients in diet products might cause allergic reactions or damage organs such as kidneys and the liver.

Furthermore, an obsession with losing weight through diet products can negatively impact mental health, leading to eating disorders. Instead of relying on these products, sustainable fat loss is best achieved through a balanced diet and regular exercise. If fat loss proves challenging, consult a healthcare provider to create a safe and effective plan.

In summary, diet products, far from being a panacea for fat loss, can harm both physical and mental health due to their problematic ingredients. Emphasizing proper nutrition and exercise remains the safest, most effective fat loss strategy.

## D for DATA

Data collection can greatly assist your fat loss journey. Regular weight tracking, either weekly or bi-weekly, can help you monitor progress and stay motivated. Whether using a traditional or smart scale, consistent checks can keep you on track.

Monitoring food intake, through a food diary or app, enables you to identify areas for healthier choices. These tools also let you track calories and macronutrient breakdowns, such as proteins, carbs, and fats.

Keep tabs on your physical activity too. Fitness trackers like smartwatches or phone apps record steps, heart rate, and other metrics, ensuring you meet daily exercise goals.

Another useful measure is recording your body dimensions. Even when the scale doesn't change, you may see progress in measurements of your waist, hips, arms, and legs. This can be done simply with a tape measure and a place to log these figures, such as a journal or app.

Don't overlook health-tracking apps and devices either. Apps like MyFitnessPal, LoseIt!, and Noom, and fitness trackers like Fitbit and Garmin, record numerous health metrics including weight, food intake, exercise, and sleep.

Lastly, consider consulting a healthcare professional. They can provide individualized guidance, body mass index (BMI), body fat percentage, and other relevant data for a safe and effective fat loss journey.

In short, tracking various health metrics and making habit adjustments based on the data can significantly aid your progress towards a healthier weight and lifestyle.

## D for DECISION

Making a decision is the catalyst that fuels change and fulfillment. It's easy to fall into the trap of self-sabotage, always pushing the transformative decision to 'tomorrow.' However, we must recognize that the power to change lies in the present moment and harness it to achieve our aspirations.

Self-care isn't just about physical well-being—it's about acknowledging our intrinsic worth and our entitlement to lead satisfying, purposeful lives. Deciding to prioritize ourselves communicates to the world that we value our own needs. But deciding is just the beginning; we must follow through with concrete actions—be it a healthier diet, a new exercise routine, or seeking support.

As we embrace change, it's crucial to practice self-compassion. There will be challenges and setbacks, but granting ourselves grace and room for mistakes helps maintain motivation and dedication to our goals.

Our decision to care for ourselves can be inspiring to those around us, sparking a ripple effect that encourages self-care and self-love. So, if you've been putting off change, it's time to act today. Prioritize personal growth and well-being, and seize the life you deserve.

Remember, you are a treasure worth cherishing. Cultivating self-love enhances the most critical relationship—the one you have with yourself. This, in turn, allows you to show up authentically for others in your life. So, take the first step today. Embrace self-care and self-love, and remember, a community of people is there to support you on your journey.

## D for DEFICIENCY

Deficiency describes a state where someone lacks a specific nutrient, such as vitamins, minerals, or other essentials, either due to inadequate intake or poor absorption.

Symptoms of nutrient deficiencies vary depending on the nutrient involved. For instance, a deficiency in vitamin C may result in scurvy, leading to fatigue and bleeding gums, while a lack of vitamin D can cause rickets, resulting in bone weakening. An iron deficiency may lead to anemia, causing fatigue, weakness, and breathlessness.

A range of factors, including poor diet, malabsorption issues, digestive disorders, or certain medical conditions, can cause deficiencies. Those following restrictive diets or with conditions impacting nutrient absorption might face a higher risk.

The typical remedy for a deficiency involves boosting intake of the deficient nutrient via dietary changes or supplements, sometimes both. In some cases, additional medical intervention might be necessary to address contributing underlying conditions.

Prevention of deficiencies is crucial for good health. Consuming a balanced, varied diet including fruits, vegetables, whole grains, lean proteins, and healthy fats is key for adequate nutrient intake. It's also vital to discuss potential nutrient deficiencies with healthcare providers, especially with a family history or other risk factors.

Remember, while deficiencies are harmful, excessive nutrient intake can also lead to health issues like liver damage from too much vitamin A, or gastrointestinal problems from excessive vitamin C. It's therefore critical to maintain a balance in nutrient intake and consult a healthcare provider before starting supplements.

To sum up, deficiencies occur when the body lacks specific nutrients, presenting diverse symptoms and causes. However, they're generally manageable via dietary changes and supplements. Balancing diet and consulting healthcare providers regarding nutrient concerns are essential.

## D for DEFY THE ODDS

"Defy the odds" symbolizes overcoming substantial obstacles and achieving what seems improbable. This can span from conquering life-threatening illnesses to rising professionally against fierce competition. It embodies tenacity, relentless determination, and the bold courage to progress despite obstacles or sacrifices.

Especially for those labeled 'overweight', 'unfit', or 'incapable', defying the odds means rejecting these stereotypes and showcasing their genuine strength and potential. The journey of fat loss isn't solely personal, it also serves as motivation for those who thought such accomplishments were unreachable.

Beyond just shedding pounds, your health journey means asserting control over your well-being and future. Implementing positive lifestyle changes can stave off chronic conditions like dyslipidemia, which increases heart disease and stroke risk due to high blood lipid levels.

Fat loss and healthier habits decrease such risks, enhancing overall health, confidence, and empowerment. Despite the challenge, remember you're not alone. A wealth of resources, from support groups to personal trainers, stand ready to aid your success.

Fat loss also positively impacts mental health, boosting self-esteem and mood, leading to greater satisfaction in all life areas. It's never too late to command your health and inspire others with your journey. By defying the odds, you not only reshape your life but also encourage others to do the same.

## D for DELAYED GRATIFICATION

In the context of healthy eating, delayed gratification—resisting immediate unhealthy temptations to meet long-term health goals—is a crucial, often underemphasized concept. This principle offers several benefits, reinforcing your commitment to long-term objectives, fostering self-discipline and willpower, and promoting a healthier relationship with food. Despite the challenges of not seeing immediate results, delayed gratification reminds you that today's healthy choices contribute to your future well-being.

Practicing delayed gratification acts as mental conditioning, teaching your brain to value long-term objectives over fleeting indulgences. Over time, this process becomes easier, transforming into a learned skill.

To foster a healthier relationship with food, breaking the cycle of poor eating habits through delayed gratification is vital. This means valuing wholesome foods and making mindful choices that help nurture a more positive attitude towards nutrition.

So how can you practice delayed gratification? Start by setting specific goals and associated non-food rewards, such as a massage or new clothing for fat loss milestones. Focusing on the long-term benefits of healthy choices, like better sleep, improved energy, and reduced disease risks, can also help deter unhealthy temptations.

In conclusion, delayed gratification is fundamental for successful dieting, encouraging motivation, building self-discipline, and developing a healthier food relationship. When unhealthy cravings arise, remember your long-term health benefits and choose delayed gratification—a skill your future self will thank you for.

## D for DETOX

Detoxification, commonly known as detox, involves purging the body of harmful substances such as toxins, chemicals, and drugs accumulated over time. This process is key for optimal health and well-being, bringing numerous benefits.

Detox enhances the digestive system by eliminating toxins that cause disruptions like bloating and constipation. It also fortifies the immune system by removing toxins that inhibit your body's natural defenses against diseases and infections.

The skin also profits from detox, as it clears toxins that cause issues such as acne and rashes, leading to healthier, more youthful skin. Detox can also increase energy levels by eliminating toxins that cause fatigue, enabling better body function.

Importantly, detox supports fat loss. Toxins can lead to weight gain and hinder fat loss efforts, but detox improves metabolism, facilitating fat loss. Additionally, it bolsters cognitive function by clearing toxins that impair mental clarity, leading to better focus and cognitive performance.

You can support detoxification with clean eating, drinking sufficient water, regular exercise, and sauna sessions. Clean eating involves consuming whole foods—fruits, vegetables, lean proteins, and healthy fats—that provide essential nutrients and help expel toxins. Water helps flush toxins from your body, while exercise and saunas promote toxin release through sweat.

In essence, detox is vital for maintaining health, benefiting various body functions. By incorporating detox strategies into your daily routine, you can boost your overall health and well-being.

You will be able to find everything you need through the following website:

https://www.the10sprotocol.com/detox

## D for DIABETES

Diabetes is a chronic ailment impacting millions globally, caused by the body's inability to produce or use insulin effectively, leading to high blood sugar levels, potentially resulting in nerve damage, kidney disease, and cardiovascular disease.

Fat loss for diabetics can be challenging but attainable with strategic steps. A low-carb diet is a good starting point as it helps maintain steady blood sugar levels. Carbohydrates turn into sugar; thus, reducing their intake can prevent blood sugar spikes.

Nutrient-dense, fiber-rich food is another vital aspect. Including vegetables, fruits, lean proteins, and healthy fats in your diet aids in blood sugar regulation and provides essential nutrients for overall health.

Physical activity is a crucial part of diabetes management during fat loss. Exercise improves insulin sensitivity, aids blood sugar control, supports fat loss, and boosts overall health.

However, it's important to remember that managing diabetes and fat loss requires professional medical guidance. Often, diabetes management involves medication, and ensuring the safety of dietary changes or exercise routines is paramount.

Other strategies for managing diabetes while losing weight include regular blood sugar monitoring, staying hydrated, and stress management. Stress can increase blood sugar levels, so techniques like meditation, yoga, or other relaxation practices are helpful.

Being well-informed about diabetes, its symptoms, and emergency responses is critical. Managing diabetes during fat loss requires a comprehensive approach involving dietary changes, physical activity, and lifestyle adjustments. With professional healthcare guidance and a balanced plan, you can achieve fat loss while maintaining healthy blood sugar levels and improving overall health.

## D for DIET

In the bustling world of diets like keto, Dukan, paleo, vegan, and more, it's easy to feel swamped when deciding which will best aid your fitness goals. These diets often target specific issues, such as fat loss or energy increase, but they may not address the fundamental factors affecting overall health and wellness.

The ABCs of Fat Loss Protocol offers a more holistic solution. Unlike other diets, it looks at not only our food habits but also our broader lifestyles, taking inspiration from the ways of our ancestors who relied on nature for their nourishment.

Modern life, heavily influenced by industrialized food systems, is marked by a surplus of processed foods rich in sugar, fats, and other unhealthy elements. The ABCs of Fat Loss acknowledges that the issues we face aren't just tied to diet, but also to our environment, lifestyle, and general health perspectives.

Using a comprehensive approach, the ABCs of Fat Loss tackles all these areas, offering a way to optimal health and wellness. It encourages a return to the lifestyle and dietary habits of our forebears, fostering the reclaiming of health in our modern context.

In conclusion, while many diets promise immediate fixes, they often concentrate on single issues. The ABCs of Fat Loss, however, provides a sustainable, all-encompassing approach. It equips you to reach your goals and experience your best health now and, in the future, in a way that aligns with the natural rhythms of life.

## D for DISEASE

Obesity, a medical condition marked by excessive body fat accumulation, can cause numerous health problems including cardiovascular disease, type 2 diabetes, certain cancers, and mental health issues. The rising global incidence of obesity poses a serious public health challenge.

Obesity elevates the risk of cardiovascular diseases, such as coronary artery disease, stroke, and heart failure. Excessive fat leads to plaque buildup in the arteries, triggering inflammation that restricts blood flow, increasing heart attack and stroke risk.

Additionally, obesity is a major risk factor for type 2 diabetes. Excessive fat impedes insulin usage, causing high blood sugar levels and associated complications like kidney disease and nerve damage. Moreover, obesity has been linked with an increased risk of certain cancers like breast, colon, and endometrial cancers. The exact reasons remain unclear, but it's suspected that excess fat cells releasing hormones can promote cancer cell growth.

Other health issues linked to obesity include sleep apnea, osteoarthritis, reproductive problems, and complications during pregnancy. Obesity can also affect mental health, leading to depression, anxiety, low self-esteem, and social stigmatization, which can in turn negatively impact academic performance, work, social interactions, and overall quality of life.

Given the undeniable connection between obesity and various diseases, it's crucial to address this issue through strategies like increasing physical activity, promoting healthy eating habits, and addressing contributing social and environmental factors. A comprehensive, multi-disciplinary approach is required to manage the health complications associated with obesity, aiming to improve individuals' and communities' health and well-being.

## D for DISCIPLINE

Discipline, the adherence to rules and principles, is a quality that can be developed over time. It is crucial for attaining goals, building beneficial habits, and making sound decisions. It embodies self-control and the determination to persist through difficulties.

Discipline encourages the formation of good habits. This is particularly crucial in areas like health and fitness where success often depends on adhering to a routine. For instance, maintaining a disciplined gym regimen increases the likelihood of reaching fitness goals.

Furthermore, discipline supports making responsible decisions by helping individuals resist impulses and carefully weigh options to make the best possible choices. In sectors like academics, sports, or business, disciplined individuals tend to excel due to their focus, organization, and resilience.

Cultivating discipline isn't a walk in the park, but it's feasible with practice. It starts with goal setting and planning, requiring self-awareness and a good grasp of personal strengths and weaknesses. Breaking down goals into manageable tasks and mapping out a timeline is essential.

Sticking to a routine and setting aside specific time for goal-related tasks is also key, as is resisting distractions. Consistency, alongside avoiding procrastination, is important. Additionally, fostering a positive mindset, focusing on the gains of discipline and rewards of goal accomplishment, and displaying patience and persistence even amidst slow progress or setbacks, is essential.

In summary, discipline is a vital trait, though challenging to master. It's about self-control, persistence, and hard work. By setting and sticking to goals, maintaining routines, and keeping a positive outlook, anyone can foster the discipline needed for success.

In order to finish, I want you to remember this: **Discipline is the strongest form of self-love. It is ignoring current pleasures for bigger rewards to come. It's loving yourself enough to give yourself all the chances to lend you future opportunities.**

## D for DOPAMINE

Dopamine, often dubbed the "feel-good" chemical, is a crucial neurotransmitter tied to our reward and motivation systems, controlling feelings of pleasure and satisfaction. It plays a key role in functions like movement, learning, attention, memory, and even fat loss, influencing our attitudes towards food and exercise.

High-fat, high-sugar foods trigger dopamine release, stimulating the brain's reward center and fueling a desire for more such foods. On the other hand, dopamine release during exercise fosters feelings of joy, promoting continued physical activity. The neurotransmitter also impacts mood and mental health, with low levels linked to depression and anxiety, and high levels of joy and contentment.

Dopamine is linked to addiction, too. Substances like cocaine, heroin, and even high-fat, high-sugar foods can stimulate dopamine release, leading to addiction-like behaviors, potential overeating, and weight gain.

In terms of fat loss, dopamine can be both beneficial, motivating healthier food choices and exercise, and detrimental, promoting addictive behaviors towards food.

Enhancing dopamine levels naturally is achievable through regular exercise and a balanced diet rich in proteins and tyrosine-containing foods, such as chicken, fish, beans, almonds, bananas, and avocados. Other dopamine-boosting activities include listening to music, spending time in nature, and connecting with loved ones. However, overeating can lead to a dopamine crash, emphasizing the importance of moderation.

Chronic stress, lack of sleep, and substance abuse can drain dopamine levels, negatively impacting overall health. Therefore, maintaining a healthy dopamine balance through exercise, a balanced diet, and other natural activities is vital for overall well-being and successful fat loss.

## D for DREAM BIGGER

Fat loss is a tough journey that involves more than just physical exertion - it demands a mental transformation and healthier attitudes towards food and self. Crucially, it requires dreaming beyond mere numbers on the scale.

Setting broader goals beyond fat loss, such as running a 5K or eating more vegetables, creates tangible targets that keep you driven and focused, even when your weight appears stagnant. Focusing on the positive changes that come with fat loss, like improved sleep and increased energy, also encourages a more upbeat perspective, enhancing your commitment to the process.

Self-care is another integral aspect of dreaming bigger. Prioritizing your needs, from getting enough sleep and hydration to indulging in enjoyable activities, reinforces both mental and physical well-being, essential for a fruitful fat loss journey.

Building a support system of friends, family, or fellow members in online communities can provide the necessary motivation and camaraderie, making the fat loss journey less lonely. Also, integrating 'cheat meals' into your diet plan in a balanced and mindful way can alleviate feelings of restriction and enhance motivation, provided they don't become a pretext for overindulgence.

In essence, dreaming bigger during your fat loss journey is a key to success. It involves setting wider goals, emphasizing positive transformations, practicing self-care, having a supportive network, and incorporating cheat meals wisely. Ultimately, successful fat loss is about more than just physical change – it's about fostering healthier relationships with food and self.

## D for DRUGS & ALCOHOL

In 2018, Alcohol was responsible for 3.3 million people. The United Nations Office on Drugs and Crime (UNODC) reports that in 2019, an estimated 585,000 people died as a result of drug use worldwide. The majority of these deaths were attributed to the use of opioids.

**All of these persons have two things in common, they all started with one drink or one shot, and they all thought they could handle their drinking or their drugs... until they couldn't.**

Drug and alcohol abuse seriously impacts a person's physical and mental health, with effects ranging from short-term to long-term. These effects vary depending on the individual, substance, consumption method, and frequency and duration of use.

Short-term effects encompass impaired judgment, distorted perception, decreased coordination, slurred speech, and impaired memory. These effects heighten the risk of accidents, injuries, and harmful behaviors like unsafe sex or overdose.

Long-term effects are more severe and include chronic health issues like liver, heart, and lung diseases. Moreover, substance abuse can trigger mental health issues like depression, anxiety, and psychosis. For young people, these effects can interfere with brain development and cause permanent cognitive deficits.

Addiction, a chronic brain disease characterized by compulsive substance seeking and use despite harmful consequences, is another significant impact of substance abuse. Changes in the brain due to addiction can affect behavior, decision-making, and judgment.

Alcohol, one of the most widely abused substances, can cause extensive damage. Heavy drinking can lead to liver inflammation, cirrhosis, liver failure, high blood pressure, heart disease, stroke, certain cancers, cognitive impairment, memory loss, and a range of mental health issues.

Drug abuse also has devastating health effects. Opioid abuse can cause respiratory depression and potentially death. Cocaine can trigger heart attacks, seizures, and strokes, while marijuana can lead to impaired memory, coordination, and judgment, as well as an increased risk of mental health problems like schizophrenia.

In conclusion, drug and alcohol abuse significantly impact physical and mental health, leading to chronic health issues, mental disorders, and addiction. Avoiding these substances is the best prevention strategy, and those struggling with addiction should seek professional help for recovery.

# E

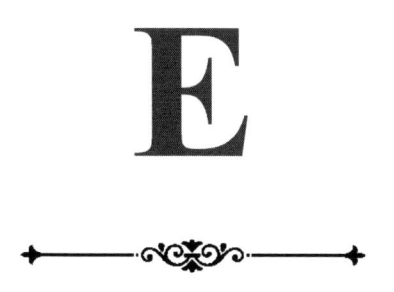

## E for EATING SPEED

Eating speed, the pace at which we consume food, is influenced by factors such as hunger, appetite, and environmental cues. However, it can have a significant impact on overall health.

Eating too fast can lead to overeating because our brains don't have enough time to register satiety. It takes about 20 minutes for our bodies to signal that we're full, so rapid eating may lead to excess calorie intake, potential weight gain, and a higher risk of health problems like diabetes and heart disease. Also, fast eating can cause digestive issues like indigestion and bloating, as it doesn't allow our system enough time for efficient food breakdown.

On the flip side, eating too slowly may lead to under-eating and potential malnutrition, and it could be frustrating and time-consuming, especially in social settings.

To foster a healthy eating speed, mindful eating is key. This involves recognizing hunger and fullness cues, choosing nutrient-dense, satisfying foods, and enjoying each bite. A useful tactic is to put down utensils between bites, allowing a few moments to chew and savor the food before continuing.

In summary, eating speed is a vital element of healthy eating. By being mindful of how quickly or slowly we eat, we can enhance digestion, avoid overeating, and maintain a healthy weight.

## E for EDUCATION

Education is a crucial element in achieving and maintaining fat loss. Often, people struggle with weight management due to a lack of understanding, resorting to fad diets that don't deliver long-term results. However, with proper education, individuals can develop lasting healthy habits.

Understanding the science of fat loss is essential, including the roles of calories, macronutrients, and metabolism. This knowledge enables people to make informed dietary decisions, aiding fat loss.

Moreover, understanding the importance of exercise in burning calories, building muscle mass, and boosting metabolism is vital. Learning about different exercise types helps integrate physical activity into daily routines.

Education also aids in cultivating healthy habits, such as preparing nutritious meals, navigating social food situations, and managing stress without resorting to comfort eating. These skills contribute to a sustainable lifestyle that supports weight management.

Structured programs providing education through nutrition and exercise classes, as well as behavioral counseling, are an effective way to learn. Alternatively, self-directed learning through nutrition and exercise literature, attending workshops, or hiring a personal trainer or nutritionist can be equally beneficial.

To sum up, education is key to successful, sustainable fat loss. By understanding the science, adopting healthy behaviors, and accessing personalized guidance, individuals can achieve their weight goals and maintain a healthy lifestyle.

## E for EGO

The ego, our self-identity, is instrumental in our health and fat loss journeys. It influences our attitudes and behaviors towards food and exercise, directly impacting goal attainment. A healthy ego promotes focus and faith in our capacity to achieve fat loss targets, whereas negative self-beliefs can obstruct progress.

To leverage the ego positively, consider the following approaches:

1. Set attainable goals: Celebrate small victories, reinforcing self-belief and spurring progress.

2. Focus on progress, not perfection: Value each step forward rather than obsessing over unattainable ideals.

3. Employ positive self-talk: Shape your ego with encouraging narratives, bolstering constructive beliefs.

4. Surround yourself with positivity: Engage with supportive individuals who reinforce your confidence.

5. Use failure as a learning experience: Rather than letting setbacks deflate your ego, see them as opportunities for growth.

It's important to remember that societal norms and media messaging can impact ego and body image, so fostering a positive self-image and healthy relationships with food and exercise is essential.

In conclusion, the ego plays a significant role in achieving fat loss goals. By setting achievable targets, celebrating progress, practicing positive self-talk, cultivating a positive environment, and learning from failures, you can harness the power of the ego. This holistic approach can lead to sustainable fat loss and overall wellness.

## E for ELECTROLYTES

Electrolytes are vital, electrically charged ions found in body fluids like blood, sweat, and urine, essential for several bodily processes. These include ensuring appropriate hydration, regulating blood pH, and conducting electrical impulses.

The primary electrolytes are sodium, potassium, calcium, magnesium, chloride, bicarbonate, and phosphate. Sodium and chloride are prevalent in extracellular fluids, potassium and magnesium are in intracellular fluids, and calcium and phosphate, primarily found in bones, are critical for muscle contractions and blood clotting.

Electrolytes are crucial for maintaining body fluid balance as they regulate water movement across cell membranes, which is critical for proper hydration. Electrolyte imbalances, such as during dehydration or excessive sweating, may lead to symptoms like muscle cramps, dizziness, and confusion.

Moreover, electrolytes are instrumental in nerve and muscle functions. Electrical impulses travel along nerve or muscle fibers by ion movement across the cell membrane, influenced by electrolyte concentration changes. Electrolyte imbalances can disrupt these electrical signals, causing muscle weakness, cramps, and irregular heartbeat.

Electrolytes also help in maintaining appropriate blood pH. If blood becomes too acidic, the body may release bicarbonate ions to neutralize excess acid.

In conclusion, electrolytes are key ions that regulate fluid balance, nerve and muscle function, and blood pH. Electrolyte imbalances can significantly impact health and often require medical attention. Hence, maintaining a proper electrolyte balance is vital for overall health and well-being.

## E for EMOTIONS

Emotional eating, a behavior where individuals use food as a coping mechanism for their emotions, significantly impacts diet and overall health. Triggered by various emotions like stress, anxiety, sadness, or boredom, individuals may eat even without hunger, often opting for foods high in sugar, salt, or fat, leading to overeating and weight gain.

Factors influencing emotional eating are manifold, encompassing past experiences with food, genetics, cultural and social impacts, and personal habits. These eating patterns can negatively affect both physical and mental health, leading to weight gain, obesity, and an increased risk of diseases like heart disease, diabetes, and cancer. It can also harm body image and self-esteem, impacting mental health.

Addressing emotional eating involves several strategies:

1. Identifying triggers: Keeping a food diary and tracking emotions helps recognize overeating triggers and gain better control over eating habits.

2. Finding alternative coping strategies: Opting for healthy ways to deal with emotions, like exercise, meditation, socializing, or engaging in relaxing activities, can help.

3. Practicing mindfulness: Techniques such as deep breathing, visualization, and meditation can assist in managing thoughts and emotions healthily.

4. Seeking support: Therapists or counselors can provide guidance and strategies to healthily manage emotions.

In conclusion, emotional eating, a common issue, can negatively affect an individual's physical and mental health. By identifying triggers, finding alternative coping strategies, practicing mindfulness, and seeking support, one can overcome emotional eating and adopt healthier eating habits.

## E for EMUNCTORY

The emunctory system comprises organs and tissues tasked with eliminating waste and toxins, crucial for maintaining our health. This system includes the skin, liver, kidneys, lungs, lymphatic system, and intestines, each playing a critical role in waste removal. The skin detoxifies through sweating, the liver filters blood, and the kidneys expel waste via urine. The lungs eliminate gaseous waste, while the lymphatic system combats infections and the intestines remove waste through bowel movements.

Malfunctioning of the emunctory system can lead to toxin accumulation, resulting in health problems such as fatigue, headaches, digestive issues, and skin problems. In severe cases, toxin buildup can lead to serious health conditions like cancer.

Maintaining the emunctory system requires a healthy lifestyle comprising a nutritious diet rich in fruits and vegetables, regular exercise, and ample water intake. Additionally, detoxification programs—like fasting, juicing, or supplements supporting liver and kidney function—can support the emunctory system, although these should be under healthcare professional guidance.

In summary, the emunctory system plays an essential role in body detoxification. Upholding a healthy lifestyle and careful use of detoxification programs under medical supervision are key for the optimal functioning of this system, ensuring overall health, and maximizing our life quality.

## E for ENDOCRINE DISRUPTOR

Endocrine disruptors are chemicals that can meddle with our endocrine system, the bodily system that regulates hormone production and release, influencing growth, metabolism, reproduction, and behavior. Interference with this system can lead to health issues like reproductive and developmental problems, cancer, and other diseases.

Endocrine disruptors can impersonate, obstruct, or interfere with the normal function of hormones, leading to wide-ranging body effects. These disruptors come from varied sources, including industrial chemicals, pesticides, plasticizers, flame retardants, and certain pharmaceuticals. They can enter our body through consumption, breathing, or skin contact, accumulating in tissues and potentially staying there for years.

Exposure to these disruptors can be particularly harmful during key developmental periods, such as fetal development and early childhood. Disruptors can interfere with the normal growth of organs and systems, potentially causing birth defects, cognitive impairment, and behavioral disorders.

Other factors like genetics, age, and overall health status can also influence the effects of endocrine disruptors. Some individuals, especially those with existing health conditions or weakened immune systems, may be more susceptible.

In conclusion, endocrine disruptors can significantly interfere with our endocrine system, affecting our health in various ways. It's important to reduce exposure to these chemicals, particularly during critical developmental stages, to safeguard our health.

## E for ENEMIES

The three foes impacting your diet and health are the processed food industry, big pharma, and your surroundings. Processed foods, filled with additives and high in calories, sugar, and sodium, contribute to obesity and other health issues. Their misleading marketing practices make healthy choices challenging. Moreover, they exploit low-income communities by offering cheaper, unhealthier options. This industry also impacts the environment negatively due to resource-intensive production and waste generation.

The pharmaceutical industry, primarily driven by profits, mainly focuses on treating symptoms rather than preventing diseases. Their business model, based on creating products that people need or desire, has raised concerns about a potential conflict of interest between generating revenue and promoting health. Critics argue the industry benefits from people staying sick, thus broadening their market.

Your social environment, while not an enemy per se, may inadvertently obstruct your health goals. Achieving a healthier lifestyle requires prioritizing your needs, acknowledging the urgency, and dedicating time and effort to your objectives. Those around you should support your journey, allowing diet-related choices, and participating in healthier activities, instead of constant socializing that could lead to dietary missteps. In sum, understanding these challenges can equip you better to tackle them and achieve your health goals.

## E for ENERGY

Fat loss often focuses on diet and exercise, but energy levels are another crucial factor often overlooked. Energy fuels our bodies and minds, motivating us to sustain healthy habits. When energy levels dip, we tend to feel sluggish, undermining our efforts towards health and fitness.

Low energy also contributes to poor sleep quality, which can further imbalance hormones, leading to increased appetite, slower metabolism, and a higher likelihood of unhealthy food choices. Hence, boosting energy is paramount for successful fat loss.

A few methods to increase energy levels include:

1. Ensuring sufficient sleep, aiming for 7-9 hours per night with quality sleep practices.

2. Engaging in enjoyable physical activities as exercise boosts energy and improves sleep.

3. Eating a balanced diet comprising whole foods, and steering clear of processed and sugary foods.

4. Staying hydrated to ward off fatigue and maintain cognitive function.

5. Managing stress through meditation, yoga, or time spent in nature.

Certain supplements and natural remedies, like moderate caffeine intake, adaptogenic herbs, and vitamin B12, can help enhance energy levels. These, however, should complement a balanced diet, regular exercise, and good sleep hygiene, not replace them.

Remember, the road to fat loss is a holistic journey that prioritizes multiple aspects of well-being, including energy levels. Adopting protocols to boost energy will improve your overall well-being, leading to more positivity and an increased capacity for physical activity. Here, it's crucial to differentiate between calories, a fuel measure, and holistic energy, which involves physical, mental, and emotional factors. By nourishing your body with nutrient-rich foods and prioritizing self-care, you can experience true vitality and reach your fat loss goals.

## E for ENTOURAGE

Achieving fat loss isn't only about counting calories or gym workouts, but it also includes considering our social and physical "entourage." Our family, friends, coworkers, and surroundings notably influence our health and fat loss journey.

Living in areas with limited fresh produce or having a sedentary job can hinder a healthy lifestyle. Moreover, social support is critical. Encouraging people can bolster our healthy habits, while negativity can obstruct our efforts.

To cultivate a supportive entourage:

1. Surround yourself with positive people who support your goals.
2. Make your surroundings conducive to health - stock nutritious food at home, have workout equipment accessible, or join a local gym.
3. Address mental and emotional health issues that might hinder healthy choices, possibly through therapy or mindfulness.
4. Seek professional help if needed, such as a nutritionist, personal trainer, or therapist.

In short, your entourage plays a pivotal role in your health and fat loss journey. Building a supportive environment and seeking needed support leads to success. Remember, the aim isn't just a number on the scale, but feeling healthy, strong, and confident.

## "YOU'RE THE AVERAGE OF THE 5 PEOPLE YOU SPEND TIME WITH"

The adage, "You're the average of the 5 people you spend the most time with," underscores the impact of social influence on our mindsets, behaviors, and lifestyle choices. Our frequent associates can shape our attitudes, beliefs, and habits—positive interactions can motivate and inspire us, while constant negativity can dampen our optimism.

The lifestyle preferences of those around us can significantly influence our own. Surrounding ourselves with health-conscious individuals often encourages similar choices, whereas exposure to harmful behaviors may lead to adopting such habits.

Consequently, it's crucial to surround ourselves with supportive people who align with our values and goals. This facilitates a nurturing environment that fosters desired habits and attitudes.

While the "average of 5" isn't a rigid rule, the role of social influence on our well-being is substantial. By being mindful of our inner circle, we can create a personal growth-friendly environment.

Consider strategizing your interactions with others whose habits don't support your goals. Manage encounters by choosing a health-conscious setting or counterbalancing with healthy choices later.

Remember, it's essential to connect with people living the lifestyle you aspire to, leveraging their energy, advice, and experiences for your growth. The goal isn't to cut ties, but to consciously choose influences that encourage personal betterment.

## E for ENVIRONMENT

The environment greatly influences our health and fat loss efforts, impacting our choices and lifestyle. Having healthy food and exercise opportunities available, along with supportive relationships, enhances the likelihood of long-term success in weight management.

Food environments sway our dietary habits. If surrounded by unhealthy options, sticking to a nutritious diet becomes tough. Conversely, easily accessible fresh produce and lean proteins encourage healthier eating.

Similarly, an environment facilitating physical activity inspires regular exercise, whereas the lack of opportunities can demotivate us. Our social circles also contribute significantly, with supportive relationships boosting morale and unsupportive ones potentially causing setbacks.

The wider environment, including access to wholesome food, exercise facilities, and potential stressors like pollution, also impacts our wellness and weight management.

Creating a beneficial environment involves several steps: modify our immediate food environment to include healthier alternatives, find enjoyable physical activities tailored to our lifestyle, lean on health-conscious friends or support groups, and advocate for health-promoting policies, such as more walking paths or healthier school meals.

In a nutshell, our environment is a potent ally in our fat loss journey. By cultivating a healthy, supportive environment -

physically, socially, and at a policy level - we can bolster our fat loss efforts, promoting holistic well-being and goal achievement.

## E for EQUILIBRIUM

Achieving fat loss revolves around balancing calorie intake with expenditure, creating a sustainable calorie deficit while ensuring adequate nutrition. The first step is a healthy, balanced diet featuring nutrient-dense foods, steering clear of extreme diets that exclude entire food groups.

Exercise is another key component, contributing to calorie burn and overall well-being. Regular, enjoyable physical activities ensure a sustainable exercise habit.

Other contributors to this balance include sufficient sleep, stress management, and avoiding overeating or emotional eating. The path to fat loss isn't linear and requires time, patience, and resilience, with each person's journey being unique.

Instead of drastic changes, making gradual alterations can ease the transition towards this balance. Small, consistent tweaks to diet or exercise habits can gradually build into a sustainable lifestyle. Also, tracking progress, including calorie intake, exercise output, weight, and body composition changes, allows for better accountability and identifies areas requiring attention.

In summary, achieving fat loss involves a balance between energy intake and output, aiming for a sustainable calorie deficit through a healthy diet and regular exercise, while considering overall health. Patience, small changes, monitoring progress, and dedication to a healthier lifestyle are vital for achieving and maintaining fat loss.

## E for EVOLVE

Evolving in the context of fat loss extends beyond diet and exercise to fostering a healthier relationship with food and body. It's about embracing growth, setting attainable goals, and acknowledging that your wellness journey is non-linear and may involve setbacks, which are learning opportunities.

Adopt a holistic wellness approach that factors in physical, mental, and emotional health. Set realistic goals, like daily workouts or incorporating more fruits and vegetables into your diet. Each small success builds momentum, reinforcing your commitment to health.

Stay open to new experiences, be it different exercise routines, healthy recipes, or mindfulness practices such as meditation. This keeps the journey interesting, maintains motivation, and aids in finding the best strategies for you.

A strong support network is key. Seek help from professionals like personal trainers or nutritionists, join a support group, or find an accountability buddy. This community provides motivation, accountability, and a safe space for sharing experiences.

Self-care and self-compassion are important, especially during setbacks. Activities like yoga, meditation, or quiet reflection can reduce stress, enhance mental and emotional health, and sustain your health journey.

In summary, evolving in fat loss involves embracing change, fostering healthier relationships with food and your body, and continuously striving to improve. Stay committed, keep a positive outlook, and appreciate the transformative journey of fat loss.

## E for EXCUSES

Making excuses can seriously impact the quality of life, fostering a lack of accountability, hindering effective communication, negatively affecting mental health, causing missed opportunities, and damaging credibility.

Excuses often enable avoidance of personal responsibility. This evasion may grant momentary relief, but it obstructs learning from mistakes, fostering repeated negative patterns and impeding personal growth.

Effective communication is also compromised when excuses dominate. People hiding behind excuses may not be truly open about their feelings and thoughts, leading to misunderstandings and conflicts, which ultimately weaken relationships and trust-building efforts.

Making excuses can be detrimental to mental health. When people use excuses to sidestep problems or fears, they risk developing anxiety, depression, and other mental health issues, stripping life of joy and meaning.

Another side effect of habitual excuse-making is the potential for missed opportunities. Excuses often prevent individuals from seizing chances that could drive personal or professional growth. This can breed regret and a sense of unfulfilled potential, diminishing life satisfaction.

Lastly, credibility can be tarnished by constant excuse-making. If seen as unreliable or untrustworthy, relationships can suffer, and opportunities may be lost, making it difficult to build a supportive network and reach personal or professional aspirations.

In summary, the negative effects of making excuses can be profound. Taking responsibility for our actions, decisions, thoughts, and feelings is vital. Being truthful with ourselves and others allows us to strengthen relationships, achieve our goals, and live a fulfilled life.

# F

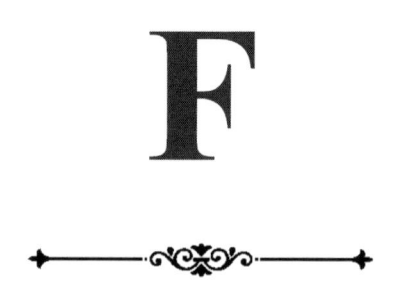

## F for FAT

## THE DIFFERENT FAT IN THE FOOD

Understanding fats in our diet is crucial for informed food choices. There are several types, including saturated, trans, monounsaturated, and polyunsaturated fats, each with different health implications.

Saturated fats, found mainly in animal products and some plant foods like coconut oil, can increase 'bad' LDL cholesterol and raise heart disease risk if consumed excessively. Trans fats, artificially hardened vegetable oils in many processed foods, can elevate LDL cholesterol, decrease 'good' HDL cholesterol, and contribute to heart disease.

Monounsaturated fats, found in olive oil and avocados, can help lower LDL cholesterol and reduce heart disease risk. Polyunsaturated fats, found in fish, seeds, and certain oils, are essential because they contain omega-3 and omega-6 fatty acids, which our bodies can't produce.

Omega-3 fatty acids can reduce inflammation, lower blood pressure, and decrease heart disease risk. Omega-6 fatty acids are beneficial in moderation, but excess can promote inflammation and increase chronic disease risk.

Remember, while the type of fat matters, quantity also counts. Overconsumption of any fat can lead to weight gain and health issues. Guidelines suggest limiting saturated fat and avoiding trans fats. Monounsaturated and polyunsaturated fats are healthier choices, but moderation is key.

In short, understanding the various types of fats helps make healthier food choices. While saturated and trans fats can be harmful, monounsaturated and polyunsaturated fats can be beneficial if consumed moderately. By selecting the right fats and monitoring portions, we can maintain a balanced, nutritious diet.

## THE EFFECT OF FAT ON YOUR HEALTH

This book shifts focus from fat loss to reducing excess body fat. Being "overweight" denotes weighing more than healthy for your height, whereas "overfat" signifies having an excessive amount of body fat. Excess fat, especially around the abdomen and organs, can cause severe health issues, even in individuals of normal weight.

Being overfat increases cardiovascular disease risks, leading to high blood pressure, elevated cholesterol, and insulin resistance. It also heightens type 2 diabetes risk, impacts insulin sensitivity, and is associated with certain cancers. Overfat individuals also face increased respiratory and joint issues, alongside mental health effects like low self-esteem and depression. Ultimately, being overfat can reduce life expectancy due to its association with chronic diseases.

Managing over fatness involves a healthy lifestyle. A balanced diet rich in fruits, vegetables, whole grains, lean protein, and healthy fats, coupled with regular physical activity, helps maintain a healthy body weight and burn excess fat. Other management strategies include regular weight monitoring, adequate sleep, and stress management through techniques like meditation or yoga. In essence, over fatness, with its linked health risks, can be prevented and managed effectively with a comprehensive lifestyle approach, boosting overall health and well-being.

You will be able to find everything you need through the following website:

https://www.the10sprotocol.com/sport

## F for FATALITY

Being overweight or obese is not an unchangeable fate. Despite obesity's complexity, influenced by genetics, hormonal imbalances, and medical conditions, it's crucial to understand that fat loss is not impossible. Consider your journey as one of self-improvement and self-care, and realize every small healthy lifestyle step matters.

A healthy diet is key to fat loss. Don't view this as deprivation, but an opportunity to nourish your body with nutrient-rich foods and limit processed ones. Likewise, see physical activity as an enjoyable routine, whether it's dancing, walking, or a new sport.

Avoid rapid-fix diets and extreme exercise routines, as these are short-term and unsustainable. Prioritize gradual, sustainable changes that become part of your lifestyle. Teaming up with a healthcare professional, like a dietitian, personal trainer, or physician, can offer personalized assistance.

Moreover, remember that fat loss also relates to emotional and mental health. Negative feelings like shame and guilt often accompany overweight individuals. Altering your mindset and self-talk is key to break from these harmful patterns and build a positive, self-loving approach towards fat loss.

In short, being overweight isn't inescapable. A positive mindset, a healthy diet, enjoyable physical activity, sustainable lifestyle changes, and self-compassion make fat loss attainable. Remember, each small healthy lifestyle step paves the way for lasting success and improved well-being.

## F for FATPHOBIA

Fatphobia, the systemic bias against overweight or obese individuals, poses severe implications for physical and mental health. This discriminatory attitude manifests in disrespectful comments, unfair job treatment, and inferior healthcare, leading to profound impacts on individuals' lives.

The media plays a significant role in fostering fatphobia by endorsing thinness as an ideal, using slim models and degrading language about overweight people. It's crucial to acknowledge that weight isn't just about "eating less"; genetics, environment, and personal habits all contribute.

Healthcare inequalities resulting from fatphobia are disturbing, with overweight people often subject to lower-quality care and bias. It's important for medical professionals to treat every patient with respect, regardless of their size.

Fatphobia is also present in workplaces, hindering overweight individuals' job prospects and promotions. This cycle exacerbates poverty and financial instability, emphasizing the need for inclusive workplace environments.

Mental health effects of fatphobia can include anxiety, depression, low self-esteem, and disordered eating, underlining the need to tackle fatphobia by challenging media stereotypes, advocating healthcare equality, and fostering body positivity. Health is multi-dimensional and weight isn't the only measure of health or worth.

The body positivity movement encourages self-love and acceptance of all body shapes, emphasizing that healthful behaviors like regular exercise and balanced diet are more important than obsessing over weight. To counteract fatphobia, we must promote respect for all bodies, challenge biases, and advocate for equality.

## EFFECTS OF FATPHOBIA

Fatphobia, the fear and discrimination against overweight people, has far-reaching consequences. It can lead to social exclusion, affecting opportunities in employment, healthcare access, and media representation, resulting in feelings of loneliness and psychological distress.

The shame associated with fatphobia can devastate self-esteem and body image, causing mental health issues. Moreover, it can trigger extreme dieting or unhealthy habits, potentially leading to serious eating disorders.

Fatphobia also contributes to healthcare disparities, as negative experiences with providers can deter overweight individuals from seeking necessary medical care, resulting in poorer health outcomes.

The discrimination and stigma from fatphobia can limit an overweight individual's ability to engage fully in society, from social events to public spaces, and can incite workplace or housing discrimination.

Another impact of fatphobia is bullying and harassment, which can lead to serious psychological issues, including depression, anxiety, and suicidal thoughts.

Finally, fatphobia fosters body shaming, in person, online, or through media, inducing feelings of shame and self-hatred.

In summary, fatphobia significantly affects the well-being of overweight individuals. It's important to realize that being overweight isn't a personal failure but a complex issue influenced by genetics, environment, and societal factors. Confronting fatphobia as a form of discrimination, and promoting body positivity and acceptance, is key to building a society that respects all body sizes.

## F for FATTY LIVER DISEASE

Fatty liver disease, a condition where excess fat accumulates in the liver, is affecting 25% of the global population. Primarily linked to poor diet and lifestyle habits, it can significantly impact fat loss goals due to:

1. Impaired Liver Function: When compromised, the liver's role in metabolizing fats and carbohydrates and filtering toxins is affected, decreasing metabolism and making fat loss difficult.

2. Insulin Resistance: This condition, linked to fatty liver disease, affects the body's glucose usage for energy and causes inflammation, complicating fat loss.

3. Hormonal Imbalances: The liver's role in regulating appetite and metabolism hormones can be disrupted, further impeding fat loss.

So, how can we support liver health and fat loss?

1. Reduce Sugar and Processed Foods: Minimizing intake of these foods, high in fructose, can support liver health.

2. Increase Fiber and Nutrient-rich Foods: Consuming fruits, vegetables, whole grains, and lean proteins can support liver detoxification processes.

3. Moderate Alcohol Intake: Limiting alcohol intake to one drink per day for women and two for men is advisable.

4. Regular Physical Activity: At least 30 minutes of moderate-intensity exercise most days of the week can promote fat loss and improve insulin sensitivity.

5. Manage Stress: Stress-management practices like meditation, yoga, or deep breathing exercises can support liver health.

In conclusion, managing fatty liver disease requires a holistic approach towards fat loss. This involves nourishing the body with nutrient-dense foods, regular physical activity, and self-care practices that support overall health.

## F for the MIRACLE of FASTING

**Fasting, also called surgery without a scalpel, is a miracle.**

Fasting, a time-honored practice spanning cultures and eras, has been used for religious, spiritual, and health reasons. Recently, its popularity has surged as an effective method for fat loss and health enhancement. It offers various significant advantages:

1. Fat loss: By using stored fat for energy, fasting (specifically intermittent fasting) facilitates weight reduction even without cutting total calorie intake.

2. Metabolic Health Enhancement: Fasting improves metabolic health by reducing insulin resistance and lowering blood sugar levels, thereby increasing insulin sensitivity.

3. Inflammation Reduction: Chronic inflammation, often a precursor to numerous diseases, can be mitigated through fasting which lowers the production of inflammatory cytokines.

4. Lifespan Extension: Although human studies are limited, fasting and calorie restriction have shown potential for lifespan extension in animal studies and may help ward off age-related diseases like Alzheimer's and Parkinson's.

5. Cognitive Function Improvement: Fasting may bolster cognitive function and shield against cognitive decline by increasing the production of brain-derived neurotrophic factor (BDNF), a promoter of new brain cell growth.

6. Heart Health Improvement: By lowering blood pressure, cholesterol, and triglyceride levels, fasting can reduce the risk of heart disease, the leading global cause of death.

7. Immune Function Enhancement: Fasting can strengthen the immune response to infections and diseases by reducing inflammation and boosting white blood cell production.

8. Spiritual Enrichment: Fasting can foster mindfulness, self-discipline, and a deeper connection to a higher power, serving as an expression of faith and commitment.

9. Cost Efficiency: As a no-cost health strategy, fasting does not require financial investment unlike medications and supplements.

10. Ease of Implementation: Fasting, encompassing various methods like intermittent fasting and alternate-day fasting, is easy to start and can be adapted to individual lifestyles.

However, before starting a fasting regimen, consulting a healthcare professional is paramount, especially for those with underlying health conditions.

Fasting stages typically include the fed state (post-meal digestion and absorption), post-absorptive state (approximately 4-6 hours after the last meal when the body starts using stored glucose and fat for energy), fasting state (after roughly 12 hours when the body relies more on fat for energy), ketosis (after around 24-48 hours when the body uses ketones from fat as alternative energy), and prolonged fasting (several days of fasting when the body starts breaking down protein for energy). The exact stages and duration may vary depending on factors like age, gender, body composition, and overall health. Prolonged fasting should only be done under medical supervision.

Common fasting methods include time-restricted feeding, alternate-day fasting, 24-hour fasting, 5:2 fasting, and extended fasting. The choice of method depends on individual health, lifestyle, and personal preferences.

Fasting can also support the body's natural detoxification processes. It facilitates the release and elimination of toxins stored in fat, stimulates autophagy (the cleaning out of damaged cells and cellular debris), and allows the body to divert energy from digestion to detoxification. While not a panacea, when done correctly and under healthcare guidance, fasting can bolster the body's innate detox mechanisms. Staying well-hydrated during a fast, aids the kidneys in eliminating toxins through urine.

**N.B.** It's important to note that water fasting is not appropriate for everyone, and it may not be suitable for individuals with certain health conditions (diabetes, people under treatment, etc.), or who are pregnant or breastfeeding. Before starting any type of fasting regimen, it's important to speak with a healthcare professional to determine whether it's safe for you.

## F for FEELINGS

Emotions significantly influence our eating habits and dietary choices. Stress prompts cravings for high-calorie, high-carb foods due to increased cortisol, a stress hormone. Countering this requires alternative stress management strategies, such as mindfulness or exercise. Boredom might induce mindless snacking as a distraction, and engaging in activities like reading or walking can help mitigate this. Feelings of sadness or depression can trigger a cycle of overeating and negative emotions, and managing these through conversation, self-care, or professional help can be beneficial. Joyful occasions or celebrations often prompt indulgence in high-calorie, nutrient-deficient foods; however, mindful eating and moderation are vital. Social situations can also impact food choices, often leading to excessive eating of calorie-dense, nutrient-poor foods, and awareness and portion control can be beneficial. Lastly, low self-esteem or negative body image can result in disordered eating, emphasizing the importance of self-care and a healthy body image. Understanding these emotional influences on our eating habits can empower us to make healthier, more mindful food choices and establish a sustainable, balanced relationship with food.

## F for FIBER

Fiber, an indigestible type of carbohydrate found in various foods, is categorized as soluble or insoluble. Soluble fiber dissolves in water, forming a gel-like substance in the intestines that aids in lowering cholesterol, regulating blood sugar, and fostering healthy gut bacteria. It's plentiful in oats, barley, beans, lentils, apples, and citrus fruits. Insoluble fiber, on the other hand, doesn't dissolve in water but adds bulk to stool, fostering regular bowel movements, and helping prevent constipation and lower colon cancer risk. It's abundant in whole grains, nuts, seeds, and the skins of fruits and vegetables.

Fiber offers numerous health benefits, including blood sugar control, cholesterol reduction, weight maintenance, and fostering feelings of fullness, which can curb overeating. It also promotes a healthy gut microbiome, crucial for overall health.

Despite the recommendation that adults consume 25-30 grams of fiber daily, many people fall short. To increase fiber intake, include a variety of fruits, vegetables, whole grains, nuts, and seeds in your diet. Drink plenty of water when increasing fiber to avoid constipation, and consider a gradual increase to prevent digestive discomfort.

## F for FOCUS

Focusing on your diet is crucial for health and wellness goals as it involves awareness of what, when, and how much you eat. Here are key reasons why it matters:

1. Better food choices: Being diet-focused enables healthier food selections. Being mindful of your intake often results in preference for whole, nutrient-dense foods over processed or high-calorie ones.

2. Portion control: By focusing on your diet, you're more likely to eat mindfully, relishing each bite, and stopping when full. This can prevent overeating and maintain calorie control.

3. Hunger and fullness awareness: Diet focus enhances understanding of your body's hunger and fullness cues, aiding in distinguishing actual hunger from eating due to boredom or stress.

4. Improved digestion: Mindful eating enhances digestion. Eating slowly and chewing food thoroughly allows for easier digestion, reduces discomfort, and optimizes nutrient absorption.

5. Motivation and accountability: Diet focus boosts motivation and accountability. Mindful eating and tracking progress helps stay aligned with health goals and keeps you motivated.

6. Stress and anxiety reduction: Being mindful and intentional about your diet can lower diet-related stress and anxiety, fostering a healthier relationship with food.

7. Better sleep and energy levels: Diet focus affects sleep and energy. A balanced, nutrient-dense diet improves energy levels and promotes better sleep.

In conclusion, diet focus is key to optimal health and nutrition. Mindful eating, choice of nutrient-dense foods, portion control, understanding hunger and fullness cues, and maintaining motivation contribute to better digestion, mental health, sleep, and energy levels. It's a cornerstone of a healthy lifestyle.

## F for FOOD

Food, with a capital F.

Food, composed of various nutrients like carbohydrates, proteins, fats, vitamins, minerals, and water, is vital for our bodies.

Carbohydrates, found in bread, pasta, fruits, etc., are a primary energy source. They're classified into simple (providing quick energy), complex (offering sustained energy), and fiber (non-digestible, aiding digestion).

Proteins are crucial for tissue growth, maintenance, and repair. These are found in foods like meat, fish, eggs, beans, and contain amino acids, some of which need dietary intake.

Fats or lipids, another energy source, are present in oils, nuts, meats, and dairy. Fats can be saturated (solid at room temperature, found in butter, cheese), unsaturated (liquid at room temperature, found in olive oil, avocados), and trans fats (created by hydrogenation, harmful to health).

Vitamins, required in minute amounts for various body functions, are either fat-soluble (A, D, E, K, stored in the body's fat cells) or water-soluble (B, C, not stored, excreted if excessive).

Minerals, also needed in small amounts, include calcium, iron, potassium, and magnesium, found in fruits, vegetables, dairy, and meats.

Water, making up around 60% of our body weight, is essential for maintaining body temperature, transporting nutrients, and waste removal. Adults should drink at least 8 cups daily.

To ensure the body gets all required nutrients, a balanced diet with variety within and across categories is crucial. Generally, a diet rich in fruits, vegetables, whole grains, lean proteins, and healthy fats ensures optimal health.

## F for FRUSTRATION

Frustration can profoundly impact diet and eating habits. Emotional eating, often a response to frustration, can lead to overeating. It's beneficial to find other methods to manage emotions, such as connecting with friends or practicing self-care. Frustration might also trigger cravings for high-fat or high-carb foods, difficult to control during stress. Recognizing these triggers and substituting them with calming activities can help manage these cravings.

In times of frustration, preparing healthy meals can seem burdensome, possibly leading to skipped meals or unhealthy food choices. Pre-planning and preparing nutritious meals can address this issue. Frustration can also lead to overeating as a form of comfort. Practicing portion control and being mindful of food choices can mitigate this.

Negative self-talk, another result of frustration, can affect self-esteem and body image, potentially leading to disordered eating. Fostering a positive body image through self-care and consuming nutrient-rich foods can help counter this. Frustration can also reduce the motivation to exercise or make healthy choices, increasing the risk of weight gain. Engaging in enjoyable physical activities and prioritizing self-care can help maintain healthy habits despite frustration. Understanding how frustration influences diet can guide us towards mindful, healthier food choices.

## F for BODY FUEL & MIND FUEL

Achieving fat loss and a healthier lifestyle necessitates a two-pronged approach that nurtures both body and mind. Body fuel, essentially the nutrients our bodies need, is a fundamental part of this. For successful fat loss, the aim is to burn more calories than consumed, which is attainable through a lower-calorie diet and increased physical activity. Understanding macronutrients like proteins, fats, and carbohydrates is essential. For instance, complex carbs from fruits, vegetables, and whole grains provide sustained energy, proteins aid muscle development and increase metabolism, and healthy fats from avocados or nuts can prevent overeating by promoting a feeling of fullness.

The other facet, mind fuel, refers to the psychological and emotional aspects of fat loss. It involves maintaining motivation for adhering to a nutritious diet and regular exercise, which can be encouraged by setting specific goals or having a workout buddy. Cultivating a positive outlook that acknowledges the benefits of a healthy lifestyle, along with a growth mindset that welcomes learning and growth, can facilitate lasting fat loss. Self-care activities like journaling, meditating, or spending time outdoors also nurture mental well-being. Balancing body and mind fuel is a key component in achieving sustainable fat loss and overall health.

# G

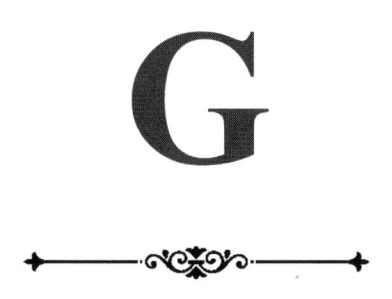

## G for GENETICS

Fat loss can often seem daunting, and genetics might play a significant role. While it can influence body type and fat storage, it's not the only determinant of weight. Even if predisposed to weight gain, remember, you're not powerless. Your lifestyle and environment, both within your control, profoundly affect your weight and health.

If genetics seem to impact your fat loss journey, seek advice from a healthcare professional or dietitian. They can help create a plan tailored to your unique needs.

Metabolism is a key factor, as it dictates how your body converts food into energy. Though genetics can affect metabolism, lifestyle, diet, and exercise play a substantial role. People with faster metabolism typically burn more calories, even when inactive.

Body composition matters, too. Individuals with more lean muscle typically burn more calories compared to those with higher body fat percentages. Hence, strength training and resistance exercises to increase lean muscle can boost metabolism and aid fat loss.

Genetics can also impact appetite and food cravings, making it harder for some to resist unhealthy foods or control portion sizes. However, this can be managed with strategies like increasing protein and fiber intake, staying hydrated, and ensuring adequate sleep.

Environmental factors like stress, lack of sleep, and exposure to toxins can also impact fat loss. Optimizing your environment to reduce these elements can aid your body's natural fat-burning processes.

In essence, while genetics do contribute to fat loss, they don't determine the outcome. A holistic approach encompassing diet, exercise, and stress management can support your body's natural fat-burning processes and help reach your goals. Remember, fat loss isn't universal; what works for one might not for another. Therefore, a personalized plan developed with a healthcare professional or dietitian can prove beneficial.

## G for GIVE UP, GIVE IN, GIVE IT ALL

When it comes to shedding weight, having a resolute mindset and readiness to make sacrifices is crucial. Here, the concepts "give up," "give in," and "give it all" become pivotal.

"Give up" signifies relinquishing unhealthy habits or foods that obstruct your fat loss journey. This could involve eliminating sugary drinks, dodging fast food, or saying goodbye to processed snacks. Breaking these habits might be challenging, but it's a vital step towards achieving your fat loss goals.

"Give in" symbolizes moderated indulgence. Allowing yourself an occasional treat is crucial, as continual denial can lead to deprivation feelings, possibly triggering binge eating. The idea is to find a balance; learn to enjoy favorite foods in moderation, while upholding a generally healthy diet.

"Give it all" implies putting your utmost effort into achieving your fat loss goals. It could mean adhering to a rigid workout routine, monitoring your food consumption, or making lifestyle changes supporting your fat loss journey. It's crucial to remain motivated and committed to your goals, particularly when the journey becomes difficult.

To effectively implement these principles, start by setting realistic goals and devise a plan of action. You might want to collaborate with a nutritionist or personal trainer to create a bespoke plan catering to your individual needs.

Remember, fat loss is a marathon, not a sprint. It requires time, patience, and consistent effort to yield results. Celebrate small victories and avoid discouragement by setbacks or plateaus.

Accountability is another significant factor in successful fat loss. Enlisting support from friends, family, or a fat loss group can boost your motivation and keep you on track. This accountability can help you remain committed when temptation lurks.

Ultimately, successful fat loss hinges on a balance between discipline and self-compassion. It's vital to stay disciplined in adhering to your plan and making healthier choices, but equally important to be forgiving when things don't go as planned. Recognize that slip-ups are part of the journey, and it's always possible to rebound.

In summary, "give up," "give in," and "give it all" are vital when embarking on a fat loss journey. By shedding unhealthy habits, indulging sensibly, and putting in maximum effort, you set yourself up for success. Stay accountable, celebrate small wins, and show yourself kindness along the journey. With commitment and a positive mindset, you can achieve your fat loss goals and enhance your overall health and well-being.

## G for GLYCEMIA

Glycemia is the concentration of glucose, a vital energy source, in our bloodstream. Originating from carbohydrates that our digestive system breaks down, glucose is absorbed into the blood and dispatched to cells for energy. Blood glucose levels are carefully managed to guarantee proper bodily function.

Stability in blood glucose levels is crucial for health. Excessively high or low glucose levels can harm the body. Elevated levels may damage blood vessels and nerves, potentially causing heart disease, kidney harm, or blindness. Conversely, lower levels might induce weakness, confusion, and dizziness, which could pose serious risks if uncontrolled.

The regulation of glycemia is a complex process involving hormones and other factors. Insulin and glucagon, produced by the pancreas, are two key hormones. Insulin lowers high glucose levels by promoting glucose absorption into cells and storing it as glycogen. Glucagon, conversely, increases low glucose levels by promoting glycogen breakdown into glucose.

Other hormones like cortisol and epinephrine also contribute to glycemia regulation. Cortisol, produced under stress, helps increase blood glucose levels. Epinephrine, or adrenaline, raises blood glucose levels by promoting glycogen breakdown and glucose production. Additionally, the liver, which produces and stores glucose, plays a crucial role in regulating glycemia.

In conclusion, glycemia, or blood glucose level, is managed by a complex system involving hormones, the liver, and other factors. Maintaining stable blood glucose levels is critical for overall health, and understanding glycemia can aid in preserving healthy blood glucose levels, thus reducing potential health issues.

You will be able to find everything you need through the following website:

https://www.the10sprotocol.com/sugar-salt

## G for GLYCEMIC INDEX

The Glycemic Index (GI) is a ranking system measuring how swiftly carbohydrate-rich foods elevate blood sugar levels. The scale goes from 0-100, with 100 being glucose. Foods with a higher GI are absorbed faster, causing a quick spike in blood sugar. Conversely, low GI foods are absorbed slowly, leading to a gradual, sustained increase in blood sugar levels.

GI depends on various factors like the type of carbohydrate, amount of fiber, presence of fat and protein, and the way the food is prepared. Simple carbs, like sugar, are digested quickly, resulting in a high GI. In contrast, complex carbs found in whole grains and vegetables digest slower, yielding a lower GI. Fat, protein, and fiber also decrease the GI by slowing carb digestion and absorption.

The GI can be a handy tool for managing diabetes. Choosing lower GI foods can help diabetics control their blood sugar and lower the risk of long-term complications. However, factors like portion sizes, meal timings, physical activity, and medication also impact blood sugar levels.

Low GI foods include non-starchy vegetables, whole grains, legumes, nuts and seeds, and low-sugar fruits. High GI foods encompass sugary drinks, refined grains, starchy vegetables, and processed snacks. In essence, GI measures how quickly a food spikes blood sugar levels, and understanding it can help in effective diabetes management.

## G for GLUTEN

Gluten, a protein in grains like wheat, barley, and rye, provides elasticity to dough and is prevalent in foods like bread, pasta, and baked goods. While it's usually safe, gluten can cause issues for those with celiac disease, non-celiac gluten sensitivity, and wheat allergy.

Celiac disease is an autoimmune condition in which gluten triggers the body to attack the small intestine, impairing nutrient absorption. Symptoms include abdominal discomfort, bloating, and fatigue. Diagnosis involves blood tests and a biopsy of the small intestine, and the only treatment is a strict gluten-free diet.

Non-celiac gluten sensitivity mimics celiac disease symptoms but lacks antibodies or small intestine damage. Its cause is unclear, but a gluten-free diet often alleviates symptoms.

Wheat allergy, an immune reaction to wheat proteins, including gluten, can cause mild to severe symptoms, potentially even anaphylaxis. Diagnosis requires skin and blood tests, and treatment involves avoiding wheat and gluten.

Gluten avoidance is key for those with these conditions, but for most, gluten is safe and can be part of a balanced diet. Despite a trend towards gluten-free diets, there's no evidence that gluten is harmful or that gluten-free diets aid fat loss for the general population. In fact, some gluten-free diets, if not carefully planned, might be less healthy, as many gluten-free products are highly processed and could be higher in sugar and fat and lower in fiber and B vitamins.

If you suspect gluten sensitivity, you might consider a gluten-free trial week to better understand your dietary needs based on your body's reactions.

## G for GOALS

Personal growth, at its core, is fueled by intense emotions originating from a myriad of experiences. Motivations can range from overcoming obstacles, fulfilling personal aspirations, or proving oneself to others. Regardless of the impetus, your quest for self-improvement is commendable, as is your commitment to self-healing.

Embarking on a journey of self-healing requires courage and resolve. It means acknowledging that something within you needs attention and care. While the process can be daunting and sometimes unsettling, the rewards are profound. In opting to heal, you're taking command of your life and embarking on a path of personal evolution and self-awareness.

Bear in mind, healing isn't a straightforward process. It's normal to face hurdles and occasional disillusionment. Yet, it's essential to keep your eye on the broader perspective and not let temporary setbacks hinder your progress. Each stride, however minuscule, leads you closer to your goal.

Approach healing with an open mind and readiness to learn. While this book and other resources provide guidance and insights, the voyage is ultimately yours. Be receptive to new perspectives, reflect on your experiences and feelings, and remember, healing is a personal journey.

What works for one may not work for another, and that's perfectly fine. Trust your intuition and focus on what resonates with you. By choosing to heal, you're making a powerful commitment to your well-being. You deserve a fulfilling and joyous life, and this journey of self-healing is a crucial step towards that objective.

## G for GOOD NEWS/BAD NEWS

I have some great news! With the ABCs of Fat Loss, you can bid adieu to unwanted fat, and not just temporarily. This unique protocol is not just about fat loss, it's also about feeling rejuvenated, vibrant, and detoxified.

But there's a catch or two. Firstly, there are no shortcuts to success, even with the ABCs of Fat Loss. You need to comprehend and follow each facet of the protocol for it to work effectively. So, be patient and give yourself time to understand and execute each step. Losing weight quickly is possible, but don't expect to consistently drop a significant amount each month. Rapid and excessive fat loss can lead to health issues like tooth and hair loss, organ dysfunction, and even cancer risk.

The second catch is that reverting to your previous unhealthy lifestyle isn't an option. Falling back into old, harmful habits will only take you back to the starting point, overweight and unwell. Therefore, it's vital to make a firm effort to avoid these detrimental behaviors and maintain a healthy lifestyle.

Success with the ABCs of Fat Loss Protocol necessitates a positive mindset, acknowledging that sustainable fat loss requires time and dedication. Remember, the perks of a healthy body are worth the effort. Understand each component of the protocol thoroughly, stay focused, and don't get disheartened by occasional setbacks.

Lastly, and most importantly, establish healthy habits for life. Integrate nutritious eating, regular exercise, and positive lifestyle decisions into your routine. By embracing a healthy lifestyle, you can maintain your fat loss and enhance your overall health.

## G for GREATNESS

Achieving greatness in fat loss means setting realistic goals and following a healthy, sustainable approach to achieve them. It's all about recognizing and using your personal strength to induce change.

The cornerstone of this journey is a powerful mindset, which means having faith in your ability to create lasting lifestyle changes, setting practical targets, staying motivated, and overcoming any obstacles that may arise.

The goal should be long-term. Rather than focusing on quick, short-lived outcomes, you should strive to establish enduring, healthy habits. Make changes to your eating habits and exercise routine that you can stick to even during challenging times.

Remember to appreciate the journey, not just the outcome. Small victories, such as resisting unhealthy snacks or finishing a tough workout, are cause for celebration and help keep you motivated.

Implementing a sound nutrition strategy is critical. This involves eating the right kinds of foods in the correct quantities. Consuming a balanced diet of lean proteins, healthy fats, complex carbs, and fruits and vegetables is crucial. Tools like food diaries or apps can help track your progress.

Physical activity is another vital piece of the puzzle. Regular exercise helps burn calories, build muscle, reduce stress, and boost mood and self-esteem.

Lastly, having a positive support system in place is key. Be it a supportive friend, a fat loss group, or a personal trainer or nutritionist. This network can provide you with motivation, guidance, and encouragement when needed.

In a nutshell, the road to greatness in fat loss involves a strong mindset, long-term focus, enjoying the journey, proper nutrition, regular exercise, and supportive company. With commitment and grit, you can make lasting changes and attain greatness.

## G for GROWTH

While fat loss is important, it should be seen as a part of a broader health and wellness approach that includes personal growth. This could mean building muscle and strength through exercises, which boosts metabolism and supports fat loss.

Moreover, growth isn't restricted to physical improvements; it also includes personal and professional development. Setting personal goals, learning new skills, or seeking career progression can be equally fulfilling and contribute to a holistic wellness journey.

Incorporating growth into your fat loss plan could involve strategies like strength training and goal setting. Strength training can come in different forms such as using weights, resistance bands, or bodyweight exercises, and it is vital for muscle development.

Setting personal goals, like learning a new language or starting a hobby, adds another dimension to your wellness journey. Achieving these targets provides a sense of purpose and enhances overall well-being.

Mental and emotional health are key facets of growth within the context of fat loss. Practices like mindfulness and stress reduction techniques can improve emotional well-being, and professional help could be sought for mental health issues like anxiety or depression.

In summary, integrating growth into your fat loss journey creates a comprehensive approach to health and wellness. The journey isn't just about shedding pounds; it's about ongoing growth and development. Prioritizing these aspects can make the journey more satisfying and successful.

# H

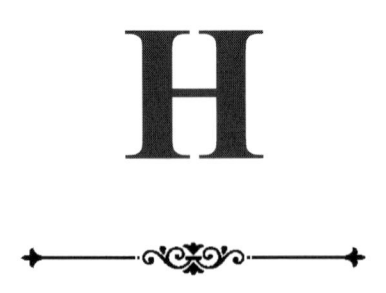

## H for HABIT

Our daily lives are structured around habits, from morning until night. These habits, either beneficial like exercising and eating healthily, or harmful like overeating or smoking, significantly influence our health and fat loss efforts. Understanding and managing these habits are key to successful fat loss.

Habits are automatic responses to environmental cues. Seeing a fast-food outlet might instantly trigger a craving for unhealthy food. Similarly, our emotional state can lead to habits, like stress-eating. These habits can either support or hinder our fat loss goals. For instance, if we habitually eat nutrient-rich foods and exercise regularly, we're more likely to succeed in losing weight. Conversely, snacking on unhealthy foods or skipping workouts can impede fat loss and lead to weight gain.

Healthy habits offer benefits beyond just fat loss. They can reduce the risk of chronic diseases such as heart disease, diabetes, and certain cancers, improve mood and mental health, and reduce stress and anxiety. They also boost energy levels, increasing productivity and overall quality of life. Furthermore, they can enhance sleep quality and quantity, contributing to better health and well-being.

In conclusion, habits play a critical role in successful fat loss and overall health improvement. Cultivating healthy habits, like regular exercise, a balanced diet, and effective stress management, can greatly support our health and fat loss goals.

## ESTABLISHING GOOD HABITS

Effective fat loss and health maintenance aren't just about short-term diets or grueling workouts. Instead, they revolve around establishing good habits and eradicating harmful ones. Here are a few tips to help you build positive habits and support your fat loss journey:

1. Set attainable and measurable goals like losing 10 pounds in three months, rather than a vague "lose weight" objective.
2. Create routines like scheduling regular workout sessions to maintain consistency.
3. Begin with small steps to avoid feeling overwhelmed. For instance, start by adding one extra glass of water to your daily intake.
4. Stay consistent. Incorporate these habits into your daily routine and stay committed.
5. Reward yourself for maintaining good habits. This practice can be motivating and help reinforce the habit.
6. Seek support from friends, family, or support groups who can understand your journey and share in your successes and challenges.
7. Be patient. Building good habits takes time. If you stumble, use it as an opportunity to learn, not a reason to quit.

Similarly, it's essential to overcome bad habits, such as mindless snacking or skipping workouts, which can hamper fat loss efforts. Here's how:

1. Identify what triggers your bad habits, and devise strategies to avoid or replace them.

2. Replace detrimental habits with healthy ones. For instance, swap mindless afternoon snacks with fruits or nuts.
3. Use positive affirmations to encourage healthy habits.
4. Surround yourself with supportive people who understand your goals.
5. Practice mindfulness to increase awareness of your actions and thoughts, which can help break bad habits.
6. If necessary, seek professional help from a dietitian or therapist to develop strategies to overcome harmful habits.

In your journey to fat loss, remember:

1. It's vital to first establish a habit, however small. The goal is not to overwhelm yourself but to get accustomed to consistently showing up every day.
2. Good habits might be tough to form but are easier to live with, while bad habits are easy to form but harder to live with. Discipline, commitment, and a willingness to change are needed to form good habits, which eventually become easy to live with. In contrast, bad habits can be detrimental to your health and wellness in the long run.
3. Tie a new habit to an existing one. This technique, known as habit stacking, reinforces consistency and makes it easier to maintain the habit.

In conclusion, long-lasting fat loss and health maintenance are a product of good habits. It's a journey that requires time and effort but can lead to healthier living in the long run.

## H for HACKS

Conquering a daunting task can be made easier by breaking it down into smaller, manageable pieces. Here's why this strategy works:

1. It curbs overwhelm. When faced with a colossal task, it's common to feel stuck. By dividing it into manageable

portions, the task becomes less intimidating and easier to start.
2. Creates a roadmap. Splitting a task gives you a plan, which keeps you organized, focused, and ensures steady progress towards your goal.
3. Fuels motivation. Facing a huge task can be demotivating. However, by splitting the task, you achieve small wins, which boosts your morale and motivates you to keep working towards the final goal.
4. Enhances prioritization. Breaking down a task makes it easier to prioritize. You can address the most critical aspects first and then move to the less crucial ones, ensuring optimal use of your time and energy.
5. Provides a clearer vision. A big task can often cloud the bigger picture. Breaking it down helps you see how each piece contributes to the whole, keeping you focused on the end goal.
6. Encourages collaboration. By dividing the task, you can assign specific parts to different team members, fostering teamwork towards a shared goal.

In conclusion, dividing a task into smaller parts reduces overwhelm, provides a clear roadmap, bolsters motivation, simplifies prioritization, offers a clearer vision, and promotes collaboration. This method helps you progress towards your goals and increases your chances of success.

However, remember that everyone makes mistakes. The key difference between successful and unsuccessful individuals is the ability to learn from mistakes and avoid repeating them. Therefore, pause, analyze your mistakes deeply, and focus on this analysis until you've eliminated these errors from your life.

## H for HAPPINESS

Happiness, a state of contentment and joy, differs from person to person due to its multifaceted nature. Some find happiness in material wealth, others in relationships or experiences, and yet others in a purposeful lifestyle. The path to happiness is individualized and varies greatly across different people.

Despite these differences, common factors contributing to happiness often include a sense of life purpose, robust social connections, good physical health, personal control over life, and resilience against adversity. Nevertheless, even with these factors in place, happiness isn't always guaranteed, indicating that it isn't a destination but an evolving, fluid journey.

Positive habits and mindsets, like gratitude, mindfulness, and self-compassion, help us appreciate the good in our lives amidst challenges and build resilience. Understanding our needs and desires and fostering positivity enhances our chance of finding everyday joy and contentment.

Becoming physically healthy is also pivotal to achieving happiness. Good physical health provides us with energy and vigor, reduces stress and anxiety, and improves mood. Physical well-being also bolsters self-confidence and self-esteem, enabling us to face new challenges enthusiastically and fostering happiness.

Moreover, physical health fosters resilience, equipping us to handle stress and recover from adversity swiftly, contributing to a sense of strength and self-efficacy. Although the path to good physical health is continuous, making small habit changes like eating healthily, exercising regularly, ensuring adequate rest, avoiding harmful habits, and getting necessary medical care can gradually improve physical well-being and enhance happiness.

In essence, the journey towards improved physical health can contribute to increased happiness. Although attaining happiness is complex and individualized, good physical health is a key element in this journey. The path towards a healthier, happier life continues with proactive steps.

## H for HASTE

In our fast-paced world, the constant rush can detrimentally affect our mental, emotional, and physical well-being. Overloading with haste leads to increased stress, causing chronic health issues like high blood pressure, heart disease, and depression. It can also decrease productivity, causing us to make mistakes and produce inferior work.

Haste strains our relationships, breeding irritability and impatience, which can lead to conflicts. It can also prevent meaningful social interactions and connections. Moreover, haste often results in impulsive decisions that may have negative consequences on our financial status, relationships, and health. It can also negatively impact our mental health, making us feel overwhelmed, anxious, and leading to exhaustion or depression.

Haste is particularly detrimental when it comes to health and fitness. Rushing into diets or unhealthy foods without introspection can impede progress. When hunger strikes, it's advisable to take a pause, breathe, and ask yourself some crucial questions: Am I genuinely hungry or is it temporary? Could I be thirsty instead of hungry? Is the food I'm craving worth it? Am I jeopardizing my efforts for short-lived pleasure? Am I in control or is the food controlling me?

Reflecting on your goals and their alignment with your current actions can prevent impulsive, unhealthy eating. If the hunger persists, engage in an activity, have a coffee with a square of dark chocolate, or cook some vegetables. By resisting the urge, you break the cycle, proving to yourself that you can control your impulses, and move closer to your goals. Repeating this process can lead to sustained health and fat loss.

## H for HEALING vs TREATING

While the words "healing" and "treating" may appear similar, they embody vastly different concepts. Healing dives into the root causes of physical or emotional issues, working to not only address symptoms but prevent future recurrences. On the other hand, treating is about managing the symptoms of a disease or condition without addressing its origin, often providing a temporary reprieve.

In today's world, health has been commodified. Some entities may profit more from chronic illness rather than wellness. A fully healed individual no longer requires ongoing care or treatments, disrupting a potential lifetime income stream. In some instances, the source of your ailment may also provide the treatment -

though not a cure - creating a perpetual demand-supply cycle, a profitable business indeed.

In creating the ABCs of Fat Loss, my focus was to dig deep into the roots of health problems. I endeavored to understand the difficulties faced by unhealthy individuals, investigating the origins of these issues, how they're dealt with, and how improvements can be made. The goal was to list these problems and provide actionable, insightful solutions to overcome them.

With the ABCs of Fat Loss, you can be sure that your health will incredibly improve and your fat percentage will drop significantly. **And remember, a patient healed is a patient lost**. Think about that.

## H for HOLISTIC

The holistic approach to medicine treats the whole person, considering their physical, emotional, mental, social, and spiritual wellness, recognizing that these aspects are interconnected and affect overall health. Instead of merely treating symptoms, this approach addresses the root cause of a problem, incorporating prevention, natural remedies, and lifestyle changes to enhance health.

Central to this approach is the belief that the body has an inherent ability to heal itself, emphasizing natural healing processes over reliance on pharmaceutical drugs or invasive procedures. It aims to identify and treat the underlying causes of diseases or conditions, rather than just managing symptoms.

Holistic medicine emphasizes personalized care, tailoring treatment plans to each patient's unique needs and circumstances. It may complement traditional treatments with therapies such as acupuncture, massage, herbal medicine, and mindfulness practices like yoga or meditation, to support natural healing processes and overall well-being.

Proactiveness is key in holistic medicine, emphasizing prevention through healthy lifestyle habits, including regular exercise, a balanced diet, and stress reduction techniques. By adopting a holistic approach to health, individuals can improve their overall well-being, reducing the risk of chronic diseases.

In summary, holistic medicine sees the person as a whole and emphasizes prevention, personalized care, and natural remedies. It addresses the root causes of health issues rather than just the symptoms. This approach can lead to improved overall health and a lower risk of chronic diseases.

## H for HOMEOPATHY

Homeopathy, an alternative medicine rooted in the concept "like cures like," suggests that substances causing symptoms in a healthy individual can help treat a sick person with similar issues. Homeopathic treatments employ highly diluted substances, believed to heighten potency despite having little to no traces of the original material. This idea, however, sparks controversy as some medical professionals doubt the effectiveness of such dilutions.

Despite the debate, homeopathy is commonly used to treat conditions like allergies, anxiety, depression, and digestive problems. Homeopaths customize treatments based on unique patient symptoms and conduct thorough consultations to develop these tailored remedies. Homeopathic solutions can be oral, topical, or injectable and come in pellets, tablets, liquids, or gels, with some available over-the-counter.

However, the scientific proof supporting homeopathy's effectiveness is scant. Few studies imply benefits, but many are small-scale or inadequately designed, which challenges the measurement of homeopathy's efficacy.

Despite these uncertainties, some people report symptom relief and enhanced well-being using homeopathy. With any healthcare approach, it's crucial to maintain an open mind and conduct comprehensive research before deciding its suitability. In sum, homeopathy, a contested yet popular treatment, requires personal investigation before adoption.

## H for HOMEOSTASIS

**This is an extremely important matter, and it's important that you treat it that way.**

Homeostasis is akin to a body's thermostat, ensuring internal stability despite external fluctuations. This key biological process in humans, much like how a home's temperature is regulated, maintains balance in the body through responses to various changes.

Several systems contribute to homeostasis. For instance, the nervous system adjusts heart rate and blood pressure, while the endocrine system, using hormones produced by various glands, aids in maintaining equilibrium. The circulatory system crucially delivers nutrients and oxygen to cells, supporting their functionality.

Homeostasis primarily focuses on upholding a stable internal environment. The body must respond to shifts in temperature, pH, and glucose levels, among others. For instance, the pancreas releases insulin to normalize rising blood glucose levels, and muscles shiver to generate heat when body temperature drops.

Nonetheless, the body's capacity to uphold homeostasis has limits. For example, exposure to extreme temperatures can cause heat stroke or hypothermia, when the body cannot adequately adjust to cool down or warm up.

Ultimately, homeostasis is essential for health and well-being. This complex process involves various systems collaborating to maintain internal stability, allowing our bodies to function effectively and stave off serious health issues. Understanding homeostasis's role is crucial, as it is a vital component of our overall health.

## H for HORMESIS

Hormesis, derived from the Greek term 'hormáein', meaning 'to excite', is the concept that controlled exposure to stressors or toxins may stimulate our body's cellular repair and adaptation mechanisms, leading to potential health and longevity benefits. This centuries-old idea has garnered renewed scientific attention in recent years with emerging evidence supporting its potential benefits.

A classic example of hormesis in action is physical exercise, a stressor that results in cellular repair and tissue growth, enhancing strength, endurance, and overall fitness. Another example is exposure to low-level toxins or radiation, which, contrary to intuition, can promote health by stimulating the body's natural defenses and prompting cellular repair. Examples of such toxins include arsenic, lead, or specific pesticides.

However, hormesis is not a universal panacea. Excessive exposure to toxins or stressors can be harmful, even fatal. But judiciously applied, it could offer significant health benefits and promote longevity. To exploit hormesis, targeted interventions can be used, such as brief periods of fasting or caloric restriction, which may stimulate hormetic pathways and promote cellular repair and adaptation. Controlled exposure to low-level radiation or toxins, as in sauna sessions or low-dose radiation therapy, may also provide health benefits.

Hormesis, an intriguing and promising concept, might hold the key to unlocking new strategies for promoting health, resilience, and slowing the aging process. Although more research is needed to fully understand hormesis's mechanisms and potential benefits, it stands as an exciting field for future scientific exploration and discovery.

## H for HORMONE

Hormones are chemical messengers, produced by glands, essential for numerous body functions including growth, mood, appetite, and metabolism. Key hormones like testosterone, estrogen, and progesterone regulate sexual development, fertility, and reproduction, while others control metabolism, stress response, immune function, and behavior. For example, cortisol, activated during stress, manages energy reserves, and insulin ensures balanced blood sugar levels.

However, hormonal balance is fragile and its disruption can greatly impact health. Imbalances may stem from genetic factors, environmental exposure, or lifestyle habits, causing conditions such as hypothyroidism, hyperthyroidism, or polycystic ovary syndrome (PCOS). Treatment for these imbalances varies from hormone replacement therapy to lifestyle changes, depending on the specific condition and its cause.

In essence, hormones are vital for our body's regulation and understanding their role is key for optimal health and disease prevention. With attentive care, we can maintain a healthy hormonal balance, promoting healthier, fuller lives.

## DIFFERENT HORMONES IN THE BODY AND THEIR ROLE

Insulin: Produced by the pancreas, insulin helps to regulate blood sugar levels by facilitating the uptake of glucose from the bloodstream into cells.

Estrogen: Produced primarily in the ovaries, estrogen is the primary female sex hormone and plays a critical role in sexual development and reproductive function.

Testosterone: Produced primarily in the testes, testosterone is the primary male sex hormone and plays a critical role in sexual development and reproductive function.

Cortisol: Produced by the adrenal glands, cortisol is released in response to stress and helps to mobilize energy reserves and prepare the body for action.

Thyroid hormone: Produced by the thyroid gland, thyroid hormone plays a critical role in regulating metabolism and growth, and development.

Growth hormone: Produced by the pituitary gland, growth hormone plays a critical role in regulating growth and development throughout the body.

Melatonin: Produced by the pineal gland, melatonin helps to regulate the sleep-wake cycle and has been shown to have antioxidant properties.

Serotonin: Produced in the brain and the digestive system, serotonin is a neurotransmitter that plays a critical role in regulating mood, appetite, and sleep.

Adrenaline (epinephrine): Produced by the adrenal glands, adrenaline is released in response to stress and helps to prepare the body for fight or flight.

Progesterone: Produced primarily in the ovaries, progesterone plays a critical role in regulating the menstrual cycle and supporting pregnancy.

Oxytocin: Produced by the hypothalamus and released by the pituitary gland, oxytocin plays a critical role in social bonding and reproductive function.

Leptin: Produced by fat cells, leptin helps to regulate appetite and energy expenditure by signaling the brain to decrease hunger and increase metabolism.

Ghrelin: Produced primarily in the stomach, ghrelin is a hormone that stimulates hunger and food intake.

Prolactin: Produced by the pituitary gland, prolactin plays a critical role in lactation and breast development.

Parathyroid hormone: Produced by the parathyroid gland, the parathyroid hormone plays a critical role in regulating calcium and phosphate levels in the body.

These are just a few examples of the many hormones that play a critical role in regulating bodily functions and processes. Hormones work in concert with one another to maintain a delicate balance within the body, and disruptions to this balance can have significant consequences for health and well-being. Understanding the role of hormones and their impact on the body is an important part of maintaining optimal health and preventing disease.

In the ABCs of Fat Loss, everything has been studied in order to optimize your balance, but overall, your production of hormones at the right time. But be patient just a little bit, we are getting there.

## H for HYPERPHAGIA

Hyperphagia, characterized by excessive hunger and overeating leading to weight gain, often complicates fat loss endeavors. It's often due to an imbalance in hormones like leptin, which signals fullness, and ghrelin, which triggers hunger. Emotional eating and sleep deprivation can also contribute, leading to increased appetite and cravings.

Managing hyperphagia involves identifying and addressing its root causes. For hormone imbalance, medical treatments can help, while therapy or counseling can tackle emotional eating by promoting healthier coping mechanisms.

To combat hyperphagia, strategies such as consuming smaller, frequent meals can help control hunger, while opting for nutrient-rich foods high in fiber and protein can enhance satiety. Practicing mindful eating, paying close attention to hunger cues, and regular exercise can regulate appetite hormones, reduce stress, and prevent overeating.

Ultimately, overcoming hyperphagia for successful fat loss demands a good grasp of its causes, implementation of effective strategies, seeking support when needed, and embracing sustainable lifestyle changes. Patience, persistence, and focusing on progress over perfection are key to this journey.

## H for HYPERSENSITIVITY

Hypersensitivity, a heightened reactivity to stimuli, can impact fat loss in various ways. Some people might react strongly to certain foods due to allergies, intolerances, or emotional associations, making it challenging to maintain a healthy diet. Others might find physical activity uncomfortable or even painful due to hypersensitivity, interfering with regular exercise, a key component of fat loss. Additionally, hypersensitivity can contribute to mental health issues, leading to stress, anxiety, and problematic eating behaviors.

Addressing these challenges requires consultation with healthcare professionals who can assist in identifying food sensitivities, adjusting workout routines, and improving mental well-being.

Customized diets, tailored exercise plans, and counseling can help manage the implications of hypersensitivity on a holistic level.

It's crucial to remember that hypersensitivity, while challenging, is a part of human diversity. Embracing it as a strength rather than a weakness can provide unique insights into health and well-being. With professional guidance and a comprehensive approach, managing hypersensitivity's challenges can lead to achieving health goals and improved overall wellness.

# I

## I for IDENTITY

Embarking on personal transformation can be daunting, yet incredibly rewarding. ABCs of Fat Loss Protocol offers more than physical fitness; it's a journey towards an overall identity overhaul. This process begins by recognizing our existing self-imposed limitations and understanding that these can change.

As you implement lifestyle changes, your perceived boundaries start to shift. You'll begin to see previously impossible goals as achievable, altering your self-perception and life vision. This transformative shift will also resonate with others, leading to a boost in your social and professional life.

Your transformed self will not be defined by limitations, but by newfound abilities and confidence. The ability to independently set and achieve goals, like running a race, will bring an unparalleled sense of accomplishment. This newfound self-reliance and motivation will fuel your journey towards better health and fitness.

Adopting new habits will facilitate an identity shift towards a disciplined, focused, and determined individual prioritizing health and well-being. This shift will permeate all aspects of your life, contributing positively beyond just physical fitness.

In sum, the ABCs of Fat Loss Protocol is a holistic personal transformation strategy. By committing to the steps and making fundamental changes, you're set on a path towards becoming a confident, self-driven individual. This journey is not merely about physical changes; it's about creating a renewed version of yourself, ready to tackle life's challenges with purpose and enthusiasm.

## I for IMAGINE

Picture this: six months to a year from now, you possess the body you've always desired. You move with ease, and things that once seemed impossible are within your reach. This vision can be an influential motivator on your journey towards health and fitness.

Visualization can be a potent tool for achieving goals. Envisioning yourself making wholesome food choices, pushing past your limits during workouts, and finally obtaining your dream body can make the process more feasible and inspiring.

The rewards of achieving fitness goals extend beyond physical transformations. It brings about a surge in self-confidence and self-esteem, instilling a sense of accomplishment. This newly acquired sense of self-assurance can pervade other aspects of your life, empowering you to face challenges with more vigor and resilience.

However, remember that reaching these goals takes time and requires dedication, hard work, and consistency. But, when you visualize the end result, it makes the journey worthwhile.

Imagine your future self, embodying your dream physique. Consider how it feels and the accomplishments you're now capable of. Use this mental image as a motivating force to remain committed to your fitness objectives. Small, consistent choices daily bring you closer to making this vision a reality. Remember, it's in your hands to take action and push yourself toward success. Keep this vision alive and remain devoted to your transformative journey. Your body is capable of incredible feats, with your vision and determination steering the way.

## I for IMPOSSIBLE

Our bodies, incredibly designed machines, are meant for action, but modern sedentary lifestyles have led to health issues. Our ancestors were active, but contemporary conveniences have made us less so, leading to muscle weakening, joint stiffening, cardiovascular problems, and chronic diseases.

Moreover, inactive lifestyles can dull our minds. The brain craves novelty and challenge, and monotony can impact our sense of purpose. Countering this requires regular physical activity - not necessarily intense gym sessions or marathon training, but simple actions like walking, climbing stairs, or light exercise.

The key is making movement habitual by linking it to existing routines. If you like morning coffee, add a few stretches while brewing. Perhaps add a quick workout during TV commercials. Pairing activities can make the new habit stick more easily.

Over time, this lifestyle change can improve energy, sleep quality, mood, and decrease chronic disease risk. Our bodies are built for movement and need it to stay robust. Don't let a sedentary lifestyle limit your potential. Link movement to an existing habit for ease. With dedication and consistency, you can transform both body and mind, leading to a healthier life. Remember, you're capable of extraordinary things, and the person to convince is you.

## I for IMMUNE SYSTEM

The immune system, our body's natural defender, interacts with fat loss in both beneficial and detrimental ways. Shedding excess fat can improve immune function by decreasing chronic inflammation linked to serious diseases like cancer, diabetes, and heart disease, and potentially enhance the function of key immune cells. However, quick fat loss or severe dieting can damage the immune system, as extreme calorie restriction might reduce immune cells' count and efficacy, thereby escalating infection risk. Maintaining immune health during fat loss requires a balanced diet filled with fruits, vegetables, whole grains, lean proteins, and healthy fats. Regular exercise, enough sleep, and stress management are equally critical. Other aspects like genetics, environmental factors, and pre-existing health conditions also influence immune function. Changes in medication usage due to fat loss can impact immune health, which underscores the importance of consulting a healthcare professional during this process. Fat loss can help boost the immune system, but it requires a careful, holistic approach that involves balanced nutrition, physical activity, good sleep, and stress management.

## I for INFLAMMATION

Inflammation is our immune system's healing response to injury or infection, but when chronic, it negatively affects health. In relation to fat loss, understanding inflammation's dual role—as both a consequence and a cause—is essential for wellness. Overabundant body fat often incites chronic inflammation, which in turn contributes to heart disease, diabetes, and certain cancers. This is because fat cells, particularly in visceral fat, emit inflammatory cytokines into the bloodstream, with levels reducing as body fat decreases, thereby diminishing inflammation.

However, fat loss can temporarily induce inflammation as the fat cell breakdown process releases inflammatory substances. Such inflammation usually subsides as the body adjusts to its new weight. But if fat loss stems from overly restrictive diets, excessive exercise, or surgical interventions like bariatric surgery, it may exacerbate inflammation.

Keeping inflammation in check during fat loss involves a balanced diet rich in anti-inflammatory foods, regular exercise, and stress management. A diet full of fruits, vegetables, whole grains, lean proteins, and healthy fats, coupled with regular exercise, can help control inflammation levels, bolster immune function, and lessen chronic disease risk.

Stress management is also critical, as chronic stress can heighten body inflammation, leading to adverse health effects such as weight gain and depression. Techniques like meditation, deep breathing, and yoga can alleviate stress, induce relaxation, and help manage inflammation.

Involving a healthcare professional in the fat loss journey is paramount, especially if existing health conditions could be affected. They can devise a personalized plan to monitor inflammation and other potential health risks.

In conclusion, while excessive body fat can induce chronic inflammation and associated health risks, fat loss may result in temporary inflammation. Holistic fat loss, emphasizing a healthy diet, regular exercise, and stress management, can mitigate this inflammation and enhance overall health.

## I for INFORMATION

In our modern era, we are bombarded with information, yet discerning useful content from redundant information is challenging, especially when it comes to fitness and wellness. The right knowledge empowers you to make insightful choices about your diet, exercise, and lifestyle, facilitating a tailored plan that resonates with your unique needs and objectives.

However, insufficient information can hinder your progress, potentially leading to ineffective or even harmful strategies, causing frustration, or prompting you to abandon your goals. Within the framework of the ABCs of Fat Loss, access to high-quality information is crucial. This program equips you with the necessary tools and knowledge to attain your desired body composition and overall health, allowing for sustainable changes that align with your long-term goals.

Remember, though, simply having access to information is not sufficient. You need to apply what you've learned, necessitating discipline, patience, and an openness to experimenting. But with the correct mindset and support, your body goals and overall happiness are achievable.

In conclusion, information is indispensable for success, particularly concerning health and wellness. By seeking out and applying quality information, you can attain the outcomes you desire, leading to a fulfilling, healthy life. Don't let an information gap limit you; instead, seize control of your health and well-being, and commence your journey towards your goals.

## I for INJURIES

Commencing a fat loss journey involves prioritizing health and safety, as potential injuries pose serious risks. They can hinder progress, thwart goals, and leave lasting physical and emotional damage. However, many injuries are preventable with the right strategy. Here are some guidelines to help safeguard against injury during your fat loss journey:

1. **Begin Gradually**: A common mistake when initiating a fat loss regimen is diving headfirst, either by drastically

cutting calories or pushing oneself excessively during workouts. This approach strains the body, increasing the injury risk. Starting slowly and gradually elevating workout intensity and calorie restriction lets your body adapt and build strength, thereby mitigating injury potential.

2. **Concentrate on Form**: Proper form during exercise is crucial to injury prevention. Focus on maintaining appropriate posture and alignment during any movement. Should you be uncertain about the correct form, consider enlisting a personal trainer or joining a class to learn the basics, thus establishing a solid foundation and decreasing injury risk.

3. **Listen to Your Body**: Listening to your body is vital in averting injuries. If you experience fatigue, soreness, or pain, pause and rest. Persisting despite discomfort can result in severe injuries over time. Understand that your body is unique and will react distinctively to different exercises and caloric restrictions, so heed its signals and adjust accordingly.

4. **Ensure Adequate Rest and Recovery**: Rest and recovery are instrumental in preventing injuries and promoting fat loss. Aim for sufficient sleep each night, as this period is when your body repairs and regenerates. Also, consider incorporating rest days into your workout schedule to allow muscle recovery.

5. **Stay Hydrated**: Hydration is paramount. Water is essential for body health and helps prevent cramps, muscle strains, and other injuries. Keep hydrated throughout the day, adding electrolytes or sports drinks if you're heavily perspiring during workouts.

Injuries can pose significant threats during a fat loss journey. However, adopting a steady approach, focusing on correct form, paying attention to your body, ensuring rest and recovery, and maintaining hydration can substantially reduce injury risks. Remember, your health and safety take precedence. If you experience discomfort or pain, don't hesitate to reassess your approach. With patience, tenacity, and an emphasis on injury prevention, you can achieve your fat loss goals while preserving your body's health and strength.

## I for INSPIRING

When you undertake a journey of self-improvement, be it physical, mental, or emotional, your transformation extends beyond just you. As you lose weight and metamorphose, you become an inspiration, embodying hope and underscoring that change is feasible and that everyone can achieve their goals. Your transformation can ignite a hopeful domino effect, inspiring others to initiate their own transformative journeys.

It isn't just about motivating others, though. As you gain confidence and feel comfortable in your own skin, you'll experience a burgeoning sense of self-pride. Recognizing that the changes weren't easy, but were undoubtedly worthwhile, you'll find yourself exuding an infectious, positive energy.

The outcome of your hard work is not merely physical, but also mental and emotional. You'll develop a strong sense of self-esteem and a conviction that you can accomplish anything. This newfound confidence and positivity will reverberate, influencing those around you positively.

Remember, the journey towards a healthier, happier self isn't solely about the destination. It's about the progressive changes, the small wins amounting to a bigger goal, and learning to love yourself and your body throughout the journey.

Embrace the transformations you're undergoing, understanding that each step towards your goal affects not only you but also those around you. When you inspire others, you create a ripple effect of positivity and hope. Ultimately, this may be the most gratifying outcome of your transformation journey.

## I for INSULIN & INSULIN RESISTANCE

Insulin, a hormone produced in the pancreas, regulates blood sugar by helping cells absorb glucose. Insulin resistance can lead to increased blood sugar, posing risks for type 2 diabetes and heart disease. It can also impede fat loss as high insulin levels discourage fat burning, favoring fat storage.

To combat insulin resistance and support fat loss:

1. Limit refined carbs: Refined carbs like white bread cause a swift surge in blood sugar and insulin. Choose whole grains, fruits, and veggies instead.

2. Consume more fiber: Fiber, an indigestible carbohydrate, decelerates glucose absorption, reducing insulin needs and promoting satiety to assist fat loss. Fiber-rich foods include whole grains, fruits, veggies, and legumes.

3. Include healthy fats: Healthy fats in nuts, seeds, avocados, and fatty fish boost insulin sensitivity and satiety, decreasing overeating.

4. Exercise regularly: Moderate-intensity exercises like walking, cycling, or swimming improve insulin sensitivity and encourage fat loss.

5. Sleep well: Adequate quality sleep enhances insulin sensitivity, while insufficient sleep increases insulin resistance. Aim for 7-9 hours nightly.

Consult a healthcare provider for an individualized plan. Some may need additional treatment, such as medication or insulin therapy. Although home insulin level tests aren't available, lab tests are important in detecting pre-diabetes, so consider requesting one from your physician.

## I for INTESTINE

Obesity significantly impacts intestinal health, leading to issues like "leaky gut," where undigested food, toxins, and bacteria escape the intestines into the bloodstream, triggering inflammation. This is more common in obese people due to chronic inflammation, changes in the gut microbiome, and alterations in gut barrier function. Obesity can also lead to non-alcoholic fatty liver disease (NAFLD), causing further intestinal damage and issues like constipation, diarrhea, and inflammatory bowel disease (IBD).

A Western diet, high in refined carbs, saturated fats, and processed foods, exacerbates intestinal damage in obesity by altering the gut microbiome and increasing inflammation. Addressing this requires lifestyle changes like diet modifications, fat loss, and sometimes medical interventions.

Left untreated, intestinal damage can result in chronic inflammation, nutrient deficiencies, autoimmune disorders, increased infection risk, liver disease, and obesity-related issues like insulin resistance, hypertension, and cardiovascular disease. Besides obesity, factors like stress, poor diet, and certain medications can also cause intestinal damage in people of healthy weight.

In short, obesity causes substantial intestinal damage due to factors like increased intestinal permeability and NAFLD. Addressing this requires dietary changes, fat loss, and potential medical interventions to improve intestinal health.

## I for FOOD INTOLERANCE

Food intolerance, a non-immune negative reaction to specific foods, can complicate fat loss. Ingesting intolerant foods can cause bloating, abdominal pain, and even skin issues, hindering fat loss. They can also lead to inflammation, disrupting blood sugar regulation, potentially resulting in insulin resistance, weight gain, and an increased risk for chronic diseases.

Detecting food intolerances is tricky due to delayed symptoms, but maintaining a food diary can help. Nevertheless, eliminating entire food groups might cause nutrient deficiencies and complicate fat loss. Thus, consulting a dietitian is crucial for maintaining a balanced diet.

Food intolerances can sometimes result from underlying conditions like celiac disease or lactose intolerance, requiring medical diagnosis and treatment. Managing these can help reduce inflammation, improve insulin sensitivity, alleviate symptoms, and increase motivation to stick to a fat loss plan.

Moreover, food intolerances can affect mental health, potentially causing mood changes, depression, anxiety, and cognitive problems, posing additional challenges to achieving fat loss goals.

In conclusion, addressing food intolerances is crucial for successful fat loss. A balanced diet guided by a dietitian, tackling underlying conditions, and managing food intolerances can boost both physical and mental health, aiding in achieving your fat loss goals.

## I for INVEST IN YOUR FUTURE

Investing in your health is about more than just immediate fat loss - it's about maintaining a healthy weight and lifestyle long-term. This requires a sustainable lifestyle and dietary changes, not quick fixes or trendy diets.

Crucially, focus on nutrient-dense, whole foods that nourish your body, keep you satisfied, and boost your energy. A balanced diet incorporating fruits, vegetables, whole grains, lean proteins, and healthy fats supports fat loss and overall health.

Combine this with regular physical activity, which benefits far beyond calorie burning, like improving heart health, strength, mood, and energy levels. Choose activities that you enjoy and can sustain.

Managing stress is also key, as it can lead to overeating and unhealthy food choices. Techniques like meditation, deep breathing, or regular massages can aid stress relief, and consequently, fat loss.

A strong support system, whether a friend, family, dietitian, personal trainer or a support group, can keep you motivated in your journey.

Remember that fat loss is a journey with ups and downs, requiring a growth mindset and focusing on progress over perfection.

To sum up, investing in your future means making lasting changes for both short-term fat loss and long-term health. By emphasizing a healthy diet, regular exercise, stress management, and a support system, you can ensure a healthier and more fulfilling future.

# J

## J for JOURNEY

Instead of viewing fat loss as an intimidating challenge, let's look at it as an adventure. By focusing on the journey rather than the destination, we can make our fat loss approach enjoyable and sustainable.

Accept that progress is unpredictable and nonlinear; there will be setbacks and hurdles. However, if we embrace these as part of our adventure, we approach fat loss with curiosity and openness.

Let's move away from obsessing over the end goal and start enjoying the process. Make healthy eating and exercise fun, not a chore. Try new recipes and workouts, shifting focus from calories and portion sizes to exploration and enjoyment.

Living in the present is crucial. Pay attention to your body's needs and cues, understanding your hunger and fullness, emotional state, and triggers impacting your eating habits.

To add excitement to this adventure, set weekly challenges. These could include trying a new healthy recipe or achieving a workout goal. Include a friend or family member for companionship and support.

Remember, fat loss is just one part of overall well-being. Adequate sleep, stress management, and cultivating healthy relationships also play a vital role in your health and happiness.

In short, envisioning fat loss as an adventure cultivates a positive, sustainable mindset. By embracing the unknown, relishing the journey, and staying present, we can make the journey fun and rewarding. After all, fat loss can be more of an exciting adventure than we think!

## J for JUICE

Vegetable juicing, combined with a healthy diet and regular exercise, can enhance fat loss efforts. It provides nutrient-dense and fiber-rich content in a low-calorie serving, allowing you to consume more vegetables than typically possible in a single meal. Consequently, it helps manage calorie intake and supports fat loss.

Drinking vegetable juice regularly can curb cravings for unhealthy, high-calorie foods. The natural sweetness of many vegetables might even help diminish sugar cravings. Additionally, it delivers health benefits beyond fat loss; its rich antioxidant content reduces inflammation and helps ward off diseases.

When preparing vegetable juice, choose a diverse mix of veggies like spinach, kale, carrots, celery, cucumber, and beets to get a broad nutrient spectrum. To enhance flavor and nutrition, add herbs such as parsley or cilantro. Avoid sweeteners as they add unnecessary calories and sugar.

Although vegetable juice aids in fat loss, it should supplement, not replace, a balanced diet comprising lean proteins, healthy fats, and complex carbohydrates.

In conclusion, vegetable juicing is a valuable addition to a fat loss regime. It provides essential nutrients and fiber with few calories, curbs unhealthy cravings, and offers additional health benefits, making it a smart choice for those aiming to improve health and well-being.

# K

## K for KNOWLEDGE

Understanding health and well-being is crucial for leading a healthy life. It enables informed choices about diet and exercise, helps identify potential health risks and methods of prevention, and aids in managing chronic conditions. Knowledge about mental health signs, symptoms, and coping mechanisms can facilitate timely intervention and emotional well-being. Additionally, knowing how to navigate the healthcare system ensures appropriate and timely care.

For instance, understanding the impact of nutritious food and effective exercises can guide you towards better dietary choices and fitness routines. If aware of your family's medical history, you can take proactive steps to mitigate potential health risks. For those managing chronic conditions, understanding the disease, its management, and knowing when to seek medical help is essential. Awareness of mental health conditions and healthy coping mechanisms, such as meditation or therapy, can aid in maintaining emotional health.

In an era where knowledge has become more accessible due to technological advancements and educational democratization, individuals have the power to educate themselves about health and well-being. The rise of the internet has opened up vast amounts of information, offering free learning across various subjects. Today, anyone with an internet connection can access education and knowledge, regardless of their financial status.

The increasing accessibility of knowledge has allowed people to explore their interests and passions, and online communities provide platforms for individuals to connect and expand their knowledge.

In conclusion, knowledge plays an indispensable role in leading a healthier life. It guides us to make healthy choices, manage chronic conditions, support mental health, and navigate the healthcare system effectively. With the democratization of education and the rise of technology, knowledge has become increasingly accessible, allowing individuals to take control of their health and well-being, explore their interests, and realize their ambitions.

# L

## L for LABEL

Understanding and utilizing food labels is pivotal for maintaining a healthy weight as they offer key details about nutritional content and ingredients, supporting informed dietary decisions. Start by noting the serving size which indicates the standard measurement and the number of servings per package. The nutritional facts correspond to one serving, so adjust accordingly if consuming more.

Calorie content per serving is vital for those aiming for fat loss as it aids in monitoring daily calorie intake. Labels also show macronutrient details - fat, carbohydrates, and protein, allowing you to tailor consumption to your dietary needs. Aim for foods low in unhealthy fats and high in unsaturated fats like nuts and fatty fish. Opt for low simple sugar, high complex carb foods for better blood sugar management.

Protein is essential for muscle building and repair, but choose sources wisely. Ingredients are listed by quantity, which helps avoid allergens or undesirable elements. Health claims on labels, such as "low fat" or "high fiber", can guide you but be cautious as some might be misleading.

In short, food labels are a vital tool for making better dietary choices, aiding in achieving and maintaining a healthy weight. However, they're just a part of the broader wellness picture.

## L for LATER

Embracing a healthy diet is essential for overall well-being, and delaying its adoption can lead to various health problems, including chronic diseases like heart disease and diabetes, nutrient deficiencies, and even mental health issues. Early implementation of a balanced diet is crucial for maintaining optimal health and mitigating these risks.

Establishing healthy eating habits can be challenging due to numerous temptations and limited knowledge about nutritious meal preparation. Yet, introducing gradual changes early on can cultivate lasting habits that promote lifelong health.

Neglecting a nutritious diet impacts not only physical health but also mental well-being, potentially leading to depression, anxiety, and impaired concentration. Prioritizing wholesome food positively affects both physical and mental health, enhancing life quality.

Moreover, postponing dietary improvements often breeds regret and frustration as reversing unhealthy habits becomes harder over time. Initiating a health-conscious diet early helps evade such regret, enabling you to enjoy the myriad benefits of balanced eating.

In conclusion, delaying a healthy diet can have negative health implications. Early adoption of such a diet, progressively adjusted, helps establish enduring habits that enhance physical and mental health, preventing chronic illnesses. So, prioritize your health and start optimizing your diet today!

## L for LAUGH

Laughter, often hailed as the best medicine, provides numerous benefits for both physical and mental well-being, fostering a healthier, more fulfilling lifestyle. Physically, laughter triggers endorphins release, acting as natural painkillers, and strengthens the immune system by enhancing antibody production and activating immune cells. This can lead to a lower susceptibility to illnesses and quicker recovery times.

On the mental health front, laughter can mitigate stress and anxiety while uplifting the overall mood, thanks to the release of happiness-associated neurotransmitters like dopamine and serotonin. Moreover, laughter strengthens social bonds, thus leading to a greater sense of happiness and fulfillment.

Intriguingly, laughter also acts as a light form of exercise, increasing heart rate and breathing, which benefits cardiovascular health. It's suggested that 15 minutes of laughter might burn calories akin to a short walk or light workout.

In times of stress or adversity, laughter can provide a relief valve, reducing tension and helping to view problems in a more positive light, thereby boosting resilience.

To sum up, laughter offers substantial physical and mental advantages, from pain reduction and immune system support to mood elevation, providing an exercise effect, and fostering resilience. To live a healthier, more joyful life, integrate laughter into your daily routine, whether through social interactions, comedies, or simply finding humor in daily life.

## L for LIFE

LIFE EXPECTANCY

The effect of fat loss extends beyond the scale, significantly influencing overall health and life expectancy. Being overweight or obese raises the risk of serious health issues like heart disease, stroke, diabetes, and some cancers, which could shorten life expectancy. Fat loss, however, can mitigate these risks and improve overall health, potentially leading to increased life expectancy. Studies suggest that even moderate fat loss (5-10% of body weight) can yield considerable health benefits.

Life expectancy is influenced not only by weight but also by lifestyle habits such as smoking, alcohol consumption, physical activity, genetics, and existing health conditions. To enhance life expectancy, adopting a sustainable approach to fat loss is key. Extreme diets or drastic calorie cuts can be detrimental to overall health and ineffective for sustained fat loss. Instead, gradual dietary and lifestyle changes, like incorporating more fruits and vegetables, reducing processed and high-fat foods, and increasing physical activity, are recommended.

Regular health screenings for early detection of health issues, along with vaccinations and other preventive measures, are also vital. To summarize, fat loss impacts not just aesthetics but also overall health and life expectancy. A sustainable approach to fat loss, focusing on overall well-being, and regular health check-ups can enhance life expectancy and health. Consultation with healthcare professionals for personalized fat loss advice is essential.

## LIFE QUALITY

Fat loss not only brings about physical improvements and reduces health risks but also significantly enhances quality of life. Excess weight can hamper daily activities, cause chronic pain, and detract from life enjoyment. Shedding this weight can improve physical function, joint health, and lessen chronic discomfort, enabling a more active and enjoyable life.

Additionally, fat loss can positively impact mental well-being. Carrying excess weight often leads to self-consciousness and low self-esteem, impairing mental health. Losing weight can elevate self-esteem, brighten life outlook, and foster greater overall satisfaction.

Improved sleep quality is another advantage of fat loss. Excess weight can lead to sleep apnea and other sleep disorders, affecting energy levels, mood, and cognitive function. Fat loss can enhance sleep quality, reduce the risk of these disorders, and promote increased energy and mental clarity.

Furthermore, fat loss can foster better social interactions. Excess weight can lead to feelings of isolation and social anxiety. However, fat loss can boost self-confidence, ease social engagement, and help form meaningful relationships, contributing to life satisfaction and overall well-being.

To maximize these benefits, a healthy, sustainable approach to fat loss is essential. Extreme diets or severe calorie restrictions can negatively impact health and are often ineffective for long-term fat loss. Instead, adopting gradual dietary and lifestyle changes like incorporating more fruits and vegetables, reducing processed and high-fat foods, and enhancing daily physical activity are recommended. Working with a healthcare professional or dietitian to develop a personalized fat loss plan can be beneficial.

In conclusion, fat loss, while commonly associated with physical improvements and reduced health risks, significantly improves overall quality of life. It can enhance physical function, mental health, sleep quality, and social interactions, contributing to a more fulfilling life. It's crucial to approach fat loss healthily and sustainably, and seek advice from healthcare professionals for personalized plans.

## L for LIPOLYSIS

Lipolysis is a critical bodily process wherein fat cells are broken down to release fatty acids and glycerol, supporting healthy weight maintenance and energy availability. When energy is required, the body primarily uses glucose from the liver and muscles. But if glucose is insufficient, it turns to lipolysis. Hormones like adrenaline and glucagon stimulate this process, triggering fat cell breakdown and releasing fatty acids and glycerol.

These components, once in the bloodstream, are transported throughout the body, providing energy for functions like muscle movement, digestion, and brain activity. This process also contributes to fat loss as the body uses stored fat for energy.

However, lipolysis requires regulation; excessive lipolysis could lead to a fatty acid buildup in the liver, potentially causing liver damage. Additionally, certain medications or medical conditions like diabetes can disrupt lipolysis, resulting in metabolic imbalances and health issues.

Promoting healthy lipolysis necessitates maintaining a balanced diet and engaging in regular exercise. A diet rich in healthy fats, protein, and complex carbohydrates can support healthy metabolism, ensuring the body has necessary nutrients for optimal function. Exercise increases energy demand and stimulates hormone release that encourages fat breakdown.

In summary, lipolysis is a vital natural process that underpins healthy weight management and ensures energy availability. While certain medications or health conditions may disrupt lipolysis, maintaining a healthy diet and regular exercise routine can promote it. Understanding lipolysis' role helps individuals take steps towards healthy metabolism, thereby maintaining optimal health and well-being.

## L for LIST

Utilizing a to-do list can be an effective tool in your fat loss journey. It helps streamline your objectives, keep you motivated, and tracks progress by breaking down your fat loss journey into manageable steps. If losing weight feels like a daunting task, a to-do list can simplify things and make the process feel less overwhelming.

This tool can also pinpoint areas of your lifestyle that need a makeover. Adding tasks like "meal prep for the week" or "evening walks" provides a clear view of daily habits that need tweaking. This method helps reveal behavior patterns contributing to weight gain and prompts healthier adjustments.

A to-do list can help you prioritize your fat loss goals. When there's a substantial amount of weight to lose, knowing where to start can be daunting. But a well-planned list can focus your efforts on impactful tasks like "eliminate sugar" or "drink more water."

Moreover, to-do lists can track your progress. During the early stages of fat loss, visible progress might be slow, but ticking off completed tasks can keep you motivated. Adding tasks like "weekly weigh-ins" or "monthly progress photos" can be helpful.

Finally, to-do lists can enforce accountability. Sharing your list with a friend or relative can provide support and keep you accountable, especially when motivation wanes or temptation kicks in. In summary, to-do lists can be powerful tools for fat loss, aiding organization, lifestyle changes, goal prioritization, progress tracking, and ensuring accountability. So, if fat loss feels overwhelming, a to-do list can keep you on track.

## L for LOBBIES

While healthcare lobbying plays a legitimate role in voicing stakeholder interests, its adverse effects can be significant when profits overshadow patient welfare.

Pharmaceutical and medical device lobbies may bend regulations, leading to the approval of untested or ineffective products, and endangering patients. Similarly, healthcare providers, insurance companies, and others can influence policy to put profits first, leading to restricted care access, decreased public health funding, and amplified health disparities.

Unethical practices like bribing officials, deceptive marketing, or manipulating scientific research can degrade public trust and the integrity of medical research, negatively affecting overall healthcare quality.

Additionally, these lobbies can drive up healthcare costs by pushing policies that favor profit over patient affordability, such as high drug prices or limited access to affordable care. These policies burden patients, particularly low-income individuals or those with chronic illnesses, by making healthcare inaccessible.

Lastly, these lobbies can obstruct progress by promoting policies favoring established players, limiting competition, and hindering the entry of innovative treatments or technologies. This stagnation harms patient health and well-being by stifling the development of new therapies.

In conclusion, while healthcare lobbying can legitimately represent stakeholders, their excessive influence can harm public health and safety by manipulating regulatory policy, engaging in unethical behavior, pushing profit-centric policies, and stifling innovation. Policymakers and the public need to remain vigilant to counteract these negative effects.

## L for LOVE

LOVE YOURSELF

Self-love is a crucial element in the fat loss journey. Instead of being driven by self-criticism, adopting a mindset of self-love and acceptance can lead to healthier lifestyle choices and more sustainable success.

Remember that your value as a person isn't tied to weight or appearance. You're inherently worthy of love and acceptance, irrespective of size. When you approach fat loss with self-love, you're more likely to make choices that nourish your body and enhance wellness, such as eating healthily, engaging in enjoyable physical activities, and adopting self-care practices.

Understand that fat loss isn't a straightforward journey; there will be ups and downs, plateaus, and setbacks. Treat these phases with self-compassion rather than criticism. Also, note that weight isn't the only measure of health. Focusing on overall health indicators like blood pressure or cholesterol levels can be more beneficial.

Self-love in your fat loss journey means taking care of yourself in a nurturing, sustainable way. If you struggle with fostering self-love, consider using daily affirmations, surrounding yourself with a supportive network, and practicing self-care activities.

In conclusion, self-love is key in your fat loss journey, encouraging healthier choices and resilience. Prioritize overall well-being overweight and allow self-love to guide you in achieving your fat loss goals and a fulfilling life.

## LOVE THE PROCESS

The journey towards fat loss should be as enjoyable as the end result. This journey is gradual, requiring love, dedication, and the ability to take joy in daily strides towards a healthier you. Savoring the process rather than solely focusing on the end goal greatly improves your odds of long-term success.

Discover physical activities that genuinely excite you, not just gym workouts. Try alternatives like dancing, hiking, or rock climbing. When you enjoy your workouts, they become a fun pastime rather than a chore, enhancing your commitment.

Food choices are also crucial. Instead of viewing dieting as a restrictive process, explore tasty, healthy alternatives. Enjoy new recipes, diverse flavors, and occasional indulgences. The goal is a balanced diet that fits your lifestyle.

Additionally, notice the mental and emotional changes. Regular exercise and balanced eating boost energy, confidence, and positivity, benefits often surpassing physical improvements.

Remember, the fat loss journey has highs and lows. Part of loving the process is accepting these fluctuations and practicing self-compassion. Don't rely solely on the scale; other health improvements may not be immediately visible.

In conclusion, savoring your fat loss journey involves taking pleasure in daily habits promoting a healthier body, enjoying exercises and meals, focusing on mental and emotional benefits, and navigating the journey's ups and downs with kindness. This approach leads to a more sustainable and successful fat loss journey.

# M

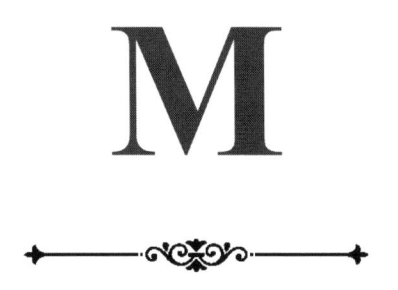

## M for MACRONUTRIENT vs MICRONUTRIENT

### MACRONUTRIENT

Macronutrients - carbohydrates, proteins, and fats - are fundamental to our health. These nutrients, required in large quantities, provide the energy needed for everyday functions.

Carbohydrates are typically the main energy source, fueling physical and mental activities. Common sources include bread, pasta, rice, and fruits. Proteins aid in tissue repair, muscle growth, immune function, and hormone production. They can be found in meats, fish, eggs, dairy, and certain plant foods.

Fats are essential for energy, brain function, hormone production, and vitamin absorption. While some fats can be harmful, others, like omega-3 fatty acids, are beneficial. Healthy fat sources include nuts, avocados, seeds, oils, and fatty fish.

Striking a balance in macronutrient intake is key, as imbalances can lead to health issues. Traditional diet guidelines may need adjustment based on personal goals and needs. For weight maintenance or fat loss, a potential balance could be 15-20% carbohydrates, 25-30% protein, and 50-60% natural non-saturated fats. This composition can aid in fat consumption, curb cravings, and enhance cognitive clarity.

Food quality is just as vital. Unprocessed, whole foods offer more nutrients and fewer additives, promoting optimal health. A nutrient-rich diet includes fruits, vegetables, whole grains, lean proteins, and healthy fats.

In conclusion, macronutrients are essential for overall health. A balanced diet featuring the appropriate amounts of carbohydrates, proteins, and fats, and quality, unprocessed foods, is key to maintaining physical and mental well-being.

## MICRONUTRIENT

Micronutrients, including vitamins and minerals, play critical roles in maintaining health. They're required in small quantities, yet they perform essential functions. Vitamins, organic compounds found in fruits, vegetables, dairy, and fortified cereals, support metabolism, growth, and development. Specific vitamin deficiencies can lead to health problems, such as scurvy, rickets, or impaired immune function.

Minerals, inorganic substances found in various foods, contribute to bone, teeth, and muscle health, and balance body fluids. For example, calcium strengthens bones and teeth, iron supports red blood cell production, zinc aids wound healing and immunity, while magnesium promotes muscle and nerve function.

Beyond preventing deficiencies, micronutrients offer additional health benefits. For instance, vitamin C acts as an antioxidant, vitamin E reduces inflammation, vitamin K assists with blood clotting, and magnesium reduces heart disease risk.

To ensure adequate intake, a balanced diet rich in nutrient-dense foods is crucial. Certain groups, such as pregnant women, seniors, and those with specific health conditions, are particularly vulnerable to micronutrient deficiencies.

In conclusion, despite being needed in small quantities, micronutrients are vital for our health. A balanced, diverse diet provides necessary micronutrients, thereby promoting overall health and preventing various health issues.

## M for MANTRA

Mantras - repetitively spoken words or phrases - can be an underappreciated yet potent ally in dieting. They can boost motivation, guide healthier choices, help overcome mental obstacles, and advocate self-care.

Dieting can be tough, particularly when progress seems slow. Mantras, such as "I am strong and capable of achieving my health goals" or "Every healthy choice I make is a step toward a happier, healthier me," can fortify motivation during these moments.

Mantras can also prompt healthier eating habits. When cravings arise, a mantra like "I choose foods that nourish my body and support my health" or "I listen to my body's signals and eat when I'm hungry, stop when I'm full," can cultivate more mindful eating.

Additionally, mantras help navigate mental hurdles. Negative self-talk and self-doubt can impede progress. Reciting "I am capable of making healthy choices and reaching my goals" or "I trust in myself and my ability to make positive changes," can overcome these barriers, fostering a more positive mindset.

Finally, mantras can promote self-care and self-love, emphasizing the importance of health and well-being. "I love and care for my body, making choices that support my health and happiness," or "I am worthy of investing time and energy into my health and well-being," can enhance self-awareness and self-compassion.

In conclusion, mantras can significantly influence dieting, bolstering motivation, supporting healthier decisions, cultivating positivity, and advocating self-care. Despite their simplicity, they can profoundly shape our mindset and overall well-being, making them a valuable tool in dietary endeavors.

## EXAMPLE OF MANTRA

There are many different mantras you can use to support your diet and overall health goals. Here are a few examples:

1. "I choose foods that nourish my body and support my health." This mantra can help you stay focused on making healthy food choices that support your overall well-being.

2. "Every healthy choice I make is a step toward a happier and healthier me." This mantra can help you stay motivated and positive, even when making healthy choices feels challenging.

3. "I trust in myself and my ability to make positive changes." This mantra can help you overcome self-doubt and limiting beliefs that may be getting in the way of your health goals.

4. "I listen to my body's signals and eat when I'm hungry, stop when I'm full." This mantra can help you tune into your body's natural signals and eat in a way that supports your health and well-being.

5. "I love and care for my body, and make choices that support my health and happiness." This mantra can help you cultivate a positive relationship with yourself and your body, and prioritize self-care in your daily life.

6. If you don't break the cycle today, you'll be doing the same mistake tomorrow

7. Break the chains of addictions, don't be a slave of your addiction

8. Believe in yourself

9. Give yourself a chance to live

10. Suffer the pain of discipline or suffer the pain of regrets

11. (My favorite) YOU CAN'T OUTRUN A BAD DIET... YOU JUST CAN'T

Remember, the most effective mantra for you will depend on your unique goals, motivations, and challenges. Experiment with different mantras and see which ones resonate with you the most.

## M for MASSAGE

While not directly related to diet, massage contributes significantly to overall well-being. This therapy manipulates the body's soft tissues, enhancing circulation, lessening muscle tension, and fostering relaxation.

A primary advantage of massage is its stress and anxiety reduction capacity. These conditions can detrimentally affect physical and mental health, leading to problems like poor sleep, weakened immunity, and heightened chronic disease risk. By lowering stress hormones and boosting serotonin and dopamine, massage can induce relaxation.

Improved circulation is another benefit of massage, crucial for the delivery of nutrients and oxygen to bodily tissues. This enhancement helps reduce inflammation, associated with health issues like heart disease, diabetes, and cancer.

Beyond its physical benefits, massage contributes to mental well-being by encouraging feelings of calm, reducing depressive and anxiety symptoms, and lifting mood. Additionally, it can relieve symptoms of chronic pain and improve the range of motion in conditions like fibromyalgia and arthritis.

Though massage isn't a direct dietary element, it forms a vital part of a healthy lifestyle. By relieving stress, promoting circulation, and inducing relaxation, massage contributes to overall health. However, it isn't a substitute for medical care, and healthcare professionals should be consulted if any pain or medical conditions exist.

In conclusion, massage's role in overall health and well-being is significant. By reducing stress, boosting circulation, and encouraging relaxation, it contributes to physical and mental health. Incorporating massage into a healthy lifestyle can unleash numerous benefits this therapy offers.

## M for MEASURE

"WHAT CAN BE MEASURED CAN BE IMPROVED"

Tracking your diet is an essential part of maintaining a healthy lifestyle, whether you're aiming for fat loss, muscle gain, or improved overall health. Using tools like calorie counting, food weighing, food diaries, and body measurements can help you understand your body better, achieve your dietary goals, and prevent frustration caused by lack of progress.

Calorie tracking ensures you're consuming the right amount of food, aligning your diet with your body's needs and objectives.

Consuming too many calories could lead to weight gain, while too few might slow down your metabolism and hinder fat loss.

Weighing food gives you an accurate understanding of what you're consuming, which is vital when aiming to lose weight or build muscle. It ensures precise macronutrient tracking, a key aspect of dietary control.

Keeping a food diary highlights your eating habits, shedding light on areas that need adjustment. Documenting each meal can reveal patterns like frequent snacking or high-calorie food consumption, enabling you to make beneficial changes.

Body measurements provide a means to monitor changes in muscle mass and body fat percentage, a motivational tool, particularly when scale numbers aren't changing.

Regularly monitoring your progress keeps you accountable, allowing you to see concrete evidence of improvement or signaling a need for changes. It fosters an understanding of your body's reactions to different foods and exercises, empowering your dietary efforts. Therefore, measurement is a key aspect of successful dieting.

You will be able to find everything you need through the following website:

https://www.the10sprotocol.com/sport and

https://www.the10sprotocol.com/satans-food-vs-superfood

## M for MENTAL

The psychological aspect of fat loss is crucial yet often overlooked. It directly affects our eating habits, activity, and lifestyle choices, with stress, self-perception, motivation, and our view of food being pivotal elements in weight management.

Stress, for instance, can lead to hormonal changes that increase appetite and sedentary behavior. Techniques like yoga, meditation, and deep breathing are beneficial in managing stress levels.

Negative self-talk can harm motivation and self-confidence, causing us to desert our diet and workout plan. Encouraging positivity through affirmations, support from loved ones, and surrounding ourselves with inspirational people can be a solution.

Motivation is critical to fat loss, but it can be fleeting. Small, attainable goals help maintain momentum, and celebrating mini victories can boost motivation. A support system, such as a workout buddy or group, brings in accountability and additional motivation.

Our perception of food plays a significant role too. People with a negative food relationship may use it as a coping tool, leading to overeating and unhealthy choices. Mindful eating and seeing food as nourishment rather than a reward or punishment can help establish a healthier food relationship.

In conclusion, addressing mental factors like stress management, positivity, goal setting, and mindful eating is key to long-term weight management success, enabling individuals to surmount mental obstacles and reach their fat loss goals.

## M for MENTAL HEALTH

Mental health significantly influences our journey towards fat loss by shaping eating habits, exercise routines, and overall motivation. Conditions such as depression, anxiety, and stress can lead to erratic eating and diminish exercise motivation, consequently hindering fat loss. Stress is particularly notorious as it triggers cortisol release, leading to increased appetite and cravings for high-calorie foods, while also disrupting sleep and impacting metabolism.

Extreme dieting or restrictive eating can lead to an unhealthy food relationship, potentially causing stress, anxiety, or depression. Therefore, improving mental health through stress management techniques like yoga, meditation, and professional help can positively affect fat loss progress.

Body image is another crucial factor. A negative body image can foster harmful behaviors like extreme dieting or over-exercising. Thus, cultivating a positive relationship with our body and food, creating a positive mindset, setting realistic goals, and focusing on progress rather than perfection are essential for achieving fat loss goals.

Additionally, a balanced, nutrient-rich diet can enhance mental health and assist fat loss. Foods rich in omega-3 fatty acids, for instance, can improve mental health. In conclusion, prioritizing mental health and overall well-being is key to successfully achieving fat loss goals.

You will be able to find everything you need through the following website:

https://bit.ly/THE10STHERAPY and

https://www.the10sprotocol.com/self-discipline

## M for METABOLISM

Metabolism, our body's system for converting food into energy, is integral to weight management and disease prevention. The rate at which we burn calories—our metabolic rate—is influenced by a variety of factors, including genetics, age, gender, body size, activity level, and importantly, our diet.

Dietary influence on metabolism comes mainly from our consumption of macronutrients: carbohydrates, proteins, and fats. Carbohydrates energize our body, but both too few or too many, especially simple sugars, can hinder metabolic efficiency. Protein, vital for tissue repair and lean muscle maintenance, supports a healthy weight. Not getting enough protein can lead to muscle loss and a slower metabolism. Fats are key for absorbing certain vitamins and maintaining healthy cell function. Yet, unhealthy fats can slow metabolism, while healthy fats can give it a boost.

Our diet also impacts metabolism via the thermic effect of food (TEF), or the energy needed to digest food. Foods with higher TEFs, like proteins, can boost metabolism, while highly processed foods and sugary drinks require less energy to digest, potentially slowing metabolism.

Diet also affects our gut microbiome, which has a crucial role in metabolism. A diet rich in fiber and complex carbs supports beneficial gut bacteria growth, improving regulation of glucose and lipid metabolism and insulin sensitivity. Conversely, a diet low in fiber and high in processed foods can disrupt gut microbiome balance and slow metabolism.

Understanding metabolism requires knowing about its two main processes: catabolism and anabolism. Catabolism breaks down larger molecules into smaller ones, releasing energy, while anabolism uses energy to create larger molecules, essential for new tissues. Balancing both processes is vital for health and preventing diseases like diabetes and obesity.

Those with a slower metabolism may struggle with weight management. Sedentary lifestyles, aging, and poor diet contribute to this. Regular exercise, strength training, and a healthy diet can help boost metabolism and support fat loss efforts. Those with a faster metabolism, burning calories more efficiently, often find it easier to maintain a healthy weight. Regular exercise and a balanced, protein-rich diet can help increase metabolic rate, making fat loss more achievable.

Understanding where you stand in terms of metabolism is crucial to weight management. Two common methods of assessing metabolic rate are visual checks and instrumental measurements. Visual checks involve observing your body's response to food intake and how quickly you gain or lose weight. Instrumental measurements can be more precise, and devices like Ketoscan provide real-time information on metabolic rate, offering personalized recommendations based on the data.

Ketoscan measures carbon dioxide levels in breath, indicating whether the body is burning carbohydrates or fat for energy. This small, portable device pairs with an app to provide personalized diet and exercise recommendations based on the user's metabolic rate. By tracking their metabolic rate, Ketoscan users can identify which foods and exercises optimize their metabolism and lead to fat loss. The app also allows users to connect with others in the Ketoscan community, fostering a supportive environment for metabolic optimization.

You will be able to find everything you need through the following website:

https://www.the10sprotocol.com/sport

## M for MICROBIOME

The microbiome, comprising microorganisms inhabiting our bodies, significantly influences our health, especially concerning diet. Key players, gut bacteria, assist in nutrient digestion and absorption, metabolism regulation, and immune function. A fiber-rich diet encourages beneficial gut bacteria, reducing inflammation and cholesterol levels and improving mental health, while a diet high in saturated fats and processed foods can disrupt this balance.

Crucially, gut bacteria impact our cravings and appetite, influencing our dietary preferences by affecting our brain chemistry. A diverse microbiome often prompts cravings for healthier foods, while a less diverse microbiome may encourage cravings for sugary and high-fat foods.

Gut bacteria also significantly influence metabolism. Certain strains produce short-chain fatty acids (SCFAs), crucial for glucose and lipid metabolism regulation, thus aiding in blood sugar level regulation and reducing risks of metabolic disorders like type 2 diabetes.

Finally, the gut microbiome also plays an essential role in immune regulation. Imbalances in gut bacteria can lead to overactive immune responses, contributing to autoimmune and inflammatory conditions. Therefore, fostering a diverse, healthy gut microbiota through a fiber-rich diet can enhance digestion, metabolism, and immune function, significantly benefiting overall health and well-being.

## M for MINDSET

Our mindset crucially impacts our diet, not only in what we eat but also in our perception and approach towards food. This necessitates a mental shift towards viewing food as nourishment, rather than categorizing it as 'good' or 'bad,' which can lead to unhealthy eating cycles and guilt.

Revamping our mindset allows us to challenge self-limiting beliefs and destructive thought patterns. Replacing negative self-talk with positive affirmations boosts confidence, self-esteem, and motivation, supporting healthier dietary choices.

A growth mindset is equally valuable, promoting a belief in our ability to improve through dedication and hard work. This mindset perceives setbacks as growth opportunities rather than failures, fostering resilience and optimism in dieting efforts.

Further, mindset adjustments can enhance body image. Embracing our bodies, prioritizing health and well-being over mere aesthetics, can alleviate body image-related stress, thereby improving quality of life.

In conclusion, reshaping our mindset is pivotal for long-term diet success. By cultivating healthier relationships with food, combating negative self-talk, endorsing a growth mindset, and bolstering body image, we can foster a supportive mentality for health goals and a healthier lifestyle. Although challenging, this mindset shift is a vital stride towards achieving dietary objectives and a healthier, happier life.

## M for MINERALS

Minerals are vital nutrients that contribute significantly to various bodily functions such as bone health, heart rate regulation, and skin health. Yet, their dietary importance often gets overlooked.

Crucial minerals like calcium, phosphorus, and magnesium help build and maintain robust bones, while zinc, copper, and manganese assist bone growth and repair. Minerals are also essential for blood pressure regulation, with potassium, magnesium, and calcium playing significant roles. Iron, zinc, and copper aid in the production of red blood cells, facilitating oxygen transport.

Minerals also contribute to skin, hair, and nail health. Selenium, zinc, and copper promote skin health, while iron enhances hair and nail health. Minerals like iron, zinc, and selenium are also essential for immune health as they aid white blood cell production. Furthermore, minerals such as chromium, magnesium, and zinc regulate our metabolism, helping convert food into energy, manage blood sugar levels, and enhance overall metabolic health.

In conclusion, minerals are indispensable nutrients that play diverse roles—from strengthening bones, regulating blood pressure, and promoting skin health, to supporting immune response and metabolic regulation. For optimal functioning, our bodies require a balanced diet rich in minerals, best obtained from mineral-rich foods like leafy greens, nuts, seeds, whole grains, and lean proteins.

## M for MIRACLE MORNING

Miracle Morning is a self-improvement strategy encouraging people to rise early and begin their day with productive routines, enhancing not only fat loss efforts but overall well-being. The idea is to wake up preferably before 6 am, allowing for better day control and reducing the sense of rush.

The morning routine should include health-enhancing activities like hydrating immediately after waking, stretching, yoga, or a walk. These practices not only facilitate fat loss but also foster overall health. The concept also emphasizes healthy eating, advising starting the day with a balanced breakfast of protein, healthy fats, and complex carbs. Avoiding processed and sugary foods in the morning helps stabilize blood sugar and curb cravings.

Besides physical activity and good nutrition, the Miracle Morning routine promotes mental and emotional self-care. This can involve activities like meditation, journaling, or reading personal development books, which can help lower stress levels and improve mental health, indirectly assisting fat loss.

Customization is a key aspect of Miracle Morning, allowing you to tailor the routine to your preferences and goals. Furthermore, it prioritizes self-care and personal growth, which often get sidelined in our busy lives.

While initially demanding, consistent practice of a Miracle Morning routine can become an integral part of your daily life, instilling control and consistency, and keeping you motivated. In conclusion, Miracle Morning, with its focus on early rising, healthy habits, physical activity, good nutrition, and self-care, can provide a supportive framework for fat loss goals and overall wellness. Its efficacy lies in patience, consistency, customization, and a positive mindset.

## M for MISTAKE

Mistakes are an integral part of the journey towards a healthy diet. While these slip-ups might initially cause discouragement, it's important to view them as growth and learning opportunities. Each mistake helps us identify what works and what doesn't in our diet plans, giving us the chance to tweak our strategies for better future choices.

Interestingly, these seemingly negative moments can boost motivation. Treating mistakes as stepping stones to success rather than setbacks encourages progress. Furthermore, navigating through dietary ups and downs helps us build resilience, preparing us to overcome challenges and reach our goals.

However, it's important to distinguish between making occasional mistakes and forming unhealthy habits. Mistakes aren't synonymous with surrendering to poor habits. Instead, they're opportunities for growth and understanding. But if we repeatedly make the same mistakes, such as frequently succumbing to cravings or making poor food choices, these can turn into difficult-to-break unhealthy habits that negatively impact our health and hinder our progress.

Repeated diet mistakes can harm self-esteem, lead to feelings of frustration and shame, and potentially cause psychological distress. Physically, continual unhealthy choices increase the risk of chronic diseases, compromising overall well-being. Therefore, proactive learning from our mistakes is essential. Reflection, pattern identification, and strategy adjustment can prevent the accumulation of errors. Seeking external support can also offer motivation and accountability.

Despite making numerous mistakes, remember it's never too late to make positive changes. Recognizing, learning from our mistakes, and adjusting our strategy can steer us towards our health goals. The frequency of our slip-ups matters too. Occasional indulgences are acceptable, but frequent unhealthy choices can become detrimental habits.

In conclusion, understanding the potential risks of accumulating diet mistakes is crucial. With proactive correction, external support, and positive lifestyle changes, we can avoid the adverse effects of frequent mistakes and successfully achieve our health goals. Remember, it's not about perfection, but persistence, resilience, and learning from our dietary journey.

## M for MONEY

The current healthcare system is more inclined towards treating illnesses rather than fostering wellness, largely due to financial incentives. This is evident in the pharmaceutical industry, where considerable profits come from selling drugs for chronic conditions, reducing the appeal of investing in preventive measures. Hospitals also earn more from treating sick patients through procedures and stays than from preventive care. However, this doesn't mean healthcare providers deliberately keep people sick; it's just how the system is structured.

This reality highlights the critical role of individuals in their health management. Embracing preventive measures like healthy eating, regular exercise, and adequate sleep can lessen chronic disease risks. Choosing healthcare providers who prioritize preventive care can also stimulate a shift towards a health-focused healthcare system.

In conclusion, despite the many providers committed to patient health, financial incentives in healthcare favor treating over preventing illness. Still, by taking charge of our health and promoting preventive care, we can contribute to a shift towards a more health-centric approach in healthcare.

## M for MOTIVATION

Motivation is the key to success in dieting, acting as the driving force to maintain discipline and consistency. It helps us resist the temptation of unhealthy foods, especially during times of stress, fatigue, or boredom, encouraging healthier choices even in tough situations.

Motivation also aids in setting realistic goals and keeping focused on them. A motivated person might set a specific fat loss target, providing a clear goal to work towards. Meeting these objectives then fuels further motivation.

Importantly, motivation fosters a positive mindset, enabling us to see setbacks as temporary obstacles rather than unmanageable barriers. This optimistic outlook motivates us to persevere in the face of challenges.

Furthermore, motivation can overcome the fear of failure. Many people hesitate to start dieting due to fear of not sticking to the diet, but strong motivation can push us past these fears, encouraging attempts and persistence.

In essence, motivation is indispensable for successful dieting. It provides the mental strength needed to resist temptations, set achievable goals, maintain a positive attitude, and conquer the fear of failure. With the right motivation, dieting becomes less daunting, and individuals are more likely to reach their goals and lead healthier lives.

## M for MORPHOLOGY

Body morphology, encompassing unique physical traits like height, weight, body composition, and metabolism, significantly influences nutritional needs. Tailoring diets according to these characteristics is key for health.

Individuals with taller heights or larger builds typically need more calories than smaller, shorter people. Similarly, those aiming for fat loss may require fewer calories compared to those maintaining their weight.

Body composition— the fat to muscle ratio—also impacts dietary needs. Individuals with higher body fat could benefit from a lower calorie, protein-rich diet to promote muscle mass and fat burn. Conversely, those with more muscle may need more calories to sustain active lifestyles.

Metabolism, the rate at which the body burns calories, is another crucial factor. People with fast metabolisms need more calories for weight maintenance, while those with slower metabolisms need less.

Body morphology can also inform food choices for health. Those with a family history of heart disease should opt for a diet low in saturated and trans fats. Meanwhile, individuals at risk of osteoporosis should focus on foods rich in calcium and vitamin D.

Dietary planning must consider individual preferences and lifestyles. For example, vegetarians or vegans need adequate plant-based protein and iron, and those with lactose intolerance should seek dairy-free alternatives high in calcium and vitamin D.

Three primary body types—ectomorph, mesomorph, and endomorph—influence nutritional needs. Ectomorphs, lean with fast metabolisms, may need more calories and protein for muscle growth. Mesomorphs, muscular with efficient metabolisms, benefit from a balanced diet, while endomorphs, rounder with slower metabolisms, might need a lower-carb diet, high in protein and healthy fats.

These body types aren't mutually exclusive; many people have traits from multiple categories. Other factors, including age, gender, and hormonal imbalances, also affect body morphology and nutritional needs, underscoring the importance of personalized meal plans created with the help of a healthcare professional or dietitian.

## M for MUSCLE

Muscle's role in diet and health is often underestimated, even though it contributes significantly to metabolic health, body composition, and overall well-being. Muscles are metabolically active, burning calories even at rest. As such, individuals with more muscle mass generally have higher resting metabolic rates, which aids in weight control. Conversely, people with less muscle mass face more challenges in fat loss due to slower metabolisms. By fostering muscle growth through a balanced diet and exercise, we can support our metabolism and improve our chances of maintaining a healthy weight.

Muscle mass also aids in refining overall body composition. Rather than focusing solely on fat loss, building and sustaining muscle mass allows us to reduce body fat and enhance lean muscle mass, boosting strength, endurance, physical function, and body aesthetics.

Importantly, strength training, vital for muscle growth, also improves bone density, mitigating osteoporosis risks, especially in women affected by menopausal hormonal shifts. The integration of strength training and muscle-building foods in our diet helps maintain robust, healthy bones.

Moreover, muscle mass correlates with lower chronic disease risks, such as type 2 diabetes, heart disease, and some cancers. Additionally, strength training can alleviate symptoms of depression and anxiety, enhancing mental health. In summary, focusing on muscle building through a nutritious diet and regular exercise is key to enhancing overall health, bolstering metabolism, improving body composition, and reducing chronic disease risk.

# N

## N for NATUROPATHY

Naturopathy is a holistic approach to healthcare, underscoring the healing power of nature and the body's intrinsic self-healing capacity. It advocates for a balanced diet rich in nutrients, ascertaining that "food is medicine". Adherents of naturopathy believe in the power of wholesome, unprocessed foods to not only prevent, but also potentially reverse disease. The diet encourages the consumption of fruits, vegetables, whole grains, lean proteins, and healthy fats, while warning against processed foods, refined sugars, and artificial additives. The primary aim is to nourish the body with appropriate nutrients to maintain health and prevent disease.

In addition to diet, naturopathy makes use of natural remedies and supplements to rectify nutritional imbalances and enhance overall health. Naturopathic practitioners may suggest dietary changes or supplements to correct deficiencies, such as lack of vitamin D or iron. They also use natural treatments like herbs, homeopathy, and essential oils to manage a variety of health issues and facilitate healing, alongside a healthy diet.

Naturopathy also prioritizes personalized care, considering each person's unique health history, lifestyle, and dietary preferences when developing a tailored nutrition plan. The focus is on addressing the root cause of health issues, rather than just treating symptoms, promoting sustainable health and preventing recurrence. To sum up, naturopathy offers an alternative route to health and wellness via diet and nutrition, advocating for balanced nutrition, natural remedies, and personalized care to not only manage symptoms, but also prevent and address underlying health issues.

## N for NEGATIVITY

Our environment, including the people, situations, and energies we engage with daily, greatly influences our physical and mental health, including our diet and lifestyle. Unrelenting negativity can discourage healthy habits and potentially lead to unhealthy eating patterns, while a positive, supportive environment can motivate healthier choices.

Persistent exposure to negative influences can spike stress levels, disrupting eating habits and potentially leading to reliance on comfort foods or overeating as coping mechanisms. Therefore, immersing ourselves in positive surroundings can reduce stress, leading to better well-being.

Furthermore, a toxic environment can disturb sleep, which impacts dietary choices. Lack of sleep is associated with increased cravings for high-sugar, high-fat foods and overeating. In contrast, a peaceful, positive environment can enhance sleep quality and promote healthier eating habits.

Lastly, constant negativity can drain energy and motivation, hampering the ability to make healthy choices. On the other hand, an uplifting, positive environment can boost motivation, making healthier choices more feasible.

It's crucial to set boundaries and distance ourselves from toxic people, passive-aggressive situations, or harmful environments. While it might not always be possible to entirely escape these situations, strategic choices can create a more peaceful existence. Prioritizing mental and emotional health by promoting positivity and kindness can dramatically improve diet and overall well-being. In short, our environment significantly impacts our diet and health, and cultivating a positive, supportive setting can result in improved eating habits and overall health.

## N for NEGOTIATION

"NEGOTIATION CAN'T BE MADE WITH YOUR WELL-BEING"

Balancing a nutritious diet with personal cravings often involves self-negotiation. This means understanding cravings as a natural part of our biology, not a failure of willpower. Managing these desires without sacrificing health goals is essential.

Planning ahead is a useful strategy for managing cravings. Preparing wholesome snacks and avoiding tempting situations, such as places with limited healthy options, can help maintain control over dietary decisions.

Setting realistic goals is vital in this process. It's impractical to completely cut out all unhealthy foods, as it can cause feelings of deprivation and potentially lead to binge eating. Instead, finding a balance between regular healthy meals and occasional treats is more sustainable.

Eating healthily should be enjoyable, not a strict discipline. Making nutritious choices most of the time while occasionally indulging in favorite foods can foster a positive relationship with food. This could include finding healthy alternatives to favored snacks, like opting for carrot sticks instead of chips when craving a crunch.

Listening to our bodies is another key aspect of self-negotiation. Our bodies often signal what they need; for instance, a sweet craving could signify a need for more carbohydrates. Fulfilling these needs with appropriate nutrients can help maintain optimal health and control cravings.

In summary, self-negotiation plays a crucial role in maintaining a balanced diet. Recognizing and managing cravings, preparing ahead, setting achievable goals, discovering healthy alternatives, and tuning in to our body's signals can help achieve a sustainable balance between satisfying cravings and upholding health goals. This approach facilitates a healthier, more enjoyable long-term eating pattern.

## N for NEUROBICS (aerobic for your neurons)

Neurobics, exercises designed to enhance cognitive function, are crucial for improving brain health and combating cognitive decline. They work by creating new neural pathways and strengthening cognition. Learning new languages, engaging in brain games, and undertaking unique activities can bolster memory and focus, particularly useful for aging individuals to help delay cognitive deterioration.

Neurobics aren't just memory enhancers, they can also help manage stress and anxiety. Participating in mentally stimulating tasks shifts our attention from stressors, reducing anxiety and promoting tranquility. Physical activities, like yoga or dancing, can also contribute to stress management and overall well-being.

Furthermore, neurobics boost creativity and problem-solving skills. Engaging in brain-stimulating tasks encourages novel thinking patterns, strengthens neural connections, and enhances our creative thinking and problem-solving capacities.

To incorporate neurobics into your lifestyle, delve into diverse mentally-stimulating activities. Consider learning new skills or hobbies, such as playing a musical instrument or painting, or engage in brain games like crosswords or Sudoku. Physical exercises that require coordination and balance, like dancing or yoga, are beneficial, as are cardiovascular activities like running or cycling that improve blood flow to the brain and alleviate stress.

In short, integrating neurobics into your daily routine can greatly enhance brain health and ward off cognitive decline, by boosting memory, focus, managing stress, and promoting creativity and problem-solving skills.

## N for NEUROMARKETING

Neuromarketing applies neuroscience to understand how the brain reacts to marketing, providing insights into consumer behavior. Yet, its use in the food industry, often to promote unhealthy food, can impact diet and health negatively.

Neuromarketing techniques can manipulate emotions, leading to unhealthy food choices. Marketers trigger our brain's reward centers through striking colors, bold fonts, and catchy phrases, thus often overriding rational decision-making and pushing us towards unhealthy options.

The widespread advertising of fast food and junk food normalizes unhealthy eating, contributing to health issues like obesity and malnutrition. Moreover, the portrayal of an idealized diet or body type can induce guilt and feelings of inadequacy, potentially leading to disordered eating and mental health issues.

Notably, neuromarketing often targets vulnerable groups, like children and individuals with mental health or addiction issues. By depicting unhealthy foods as fun and attractive, children are drawn in. Similarly, individuals with addiction or mental health issues are more susceptible to the manipulation of their reward centers, making unhealthy choices harder to resist.

While neuromarketing provides important consumer insights, awareness of its potential harm is crucial. Recognizing manipulative techniques and being mindful of our impulses can support healthier choices. Regulatory measures limiting neuromarketing's negative impact and promoting accurate, unbiased nutritional information are also vital. Awareness of triggers for unhealthy food cravings can empower individuals to make healthier decisions. REMEMBER, YOUR HEALTH IS YOUR RESPONSIBILITY, AND PROTECTING IT SHOULD BE YOUR UTMOST PRIORITY.

## N for NEUROSCIENCE

Neuroscience has enriched our comprehension of nutrition by illuminating how diet affects the brain. It has identified "brain foods," such as omega-3 fatty acids, antioxidants, and complex carbohydrates, as essential for brain health, enhancing cognitive function, memory, and mood.

The field has also revealed how foods high in sugar and fat stimulate the brain's reward circuits, similar to addictive substances. This understanding aids in making healthier food choices and avoiding overeating.

Neuroscience has further explored the relationship between stress and diet. Chronic stress can disrupt physical and mental health, leading to unhealthy eating habits by affecting the hypothalamic-pituitary-adrenal (HPA) axis that regulates appetite, cravings, and metabolism.

Moreover, neuroscience has elucidated the gut-brain axis's significance, showcasing the crucial connection between our gut microbiome, appetite, digestion, and mood. This understanding has spurred the rise of "nutritional psychiatry," a field studying nutrition's impact on mental health.

In essence, neuroscience offers valuable insights into the intricate connection between our diet and brain. It encourages healthier food choices, stress management, and attention to gut health. Applying these findings can help us lead healthier and more fulfilled lives.

## N for NEXT MEAL

Planning and prepping meals in advance can greatly contribute to maintaining a healthy diet. Being ready for the next meal removes the stress of last-minute decisions, which often lead to unhealthy choices. A pre-arranged meal offers a healthier alternative to convenient but nutrient-poor food, aligning with our health goals.

Pre-prepared meals also save time and money. Bulk buying and cooking in advance streamline our daily routine, while resisting the temptation of expensive dining out or takeout thanks to a ready meal brings financial benefits.

Staying consistent with diet plans is easier when meals are prepared ahead. This routine fosters long-term healthy eating habits, even in stressful situations. Meal prep, an approach involving preparing meals or parts of meals ahead of time, can also serve as a creative outlet, with opportunities to experiment with new recipes.

Packing a wholesome lunch for work is another effective strategy. It not only ensures a healthy choice but also saves money and curbs the impulse to eat out.

In short, planning and preparing meals in advance is a pivotal strategy for a healthy diet, offering advantages like wise decisions, prevention of unhealthy choices, time and money savings, adherence to dietary goals, and an element of culinary creativity. Having the next meal ready can make healthy eating a consistent and enjoyable part of our lives.

## N for LEARNING TO SAY NO

### IN GENERAL

Saying 'no' can be tough given our natural inclination to be obliging and liked. Yet, mastering the ability to say 'no' is critical in setting healthy boundaries, prioritizing our needs, and meeting goals.

By saying 'no', we set essential boundaries that prevent feelings of overwhelm or exploitation, facilitating balanced relationships. It's a means to cap what we accept, allowing us to focus on our own needs.

Saying 'no' also represents self-care. We often put others before ourselves, neglecting our well-being. When we're feeling stressed or drained, saying 'no' provides us a chance to recharge and prioritize our mental wellness.

Moreover, saying 'no' keeps us aligned with our objectives. Accepting every request can distract us from our priorities. For example, declining social engagements when preparing for an important test allows us to optimize our study time.

Saying 'no' can boost our self-esteem. Regularly saying 'yes' can make us feel out of control, while saying 'no' helps us regain control, assert ourselves positively, and strengthens confidence in our decision-making.

Lastly, saying 'no' contributes to honesty and authenticity in relationships. Agreeing to things unwillingly can lead to resentment. Conversely, saying 'no' fosters truthful communication and respect in relationships.

In essence, learning to say 'no' is a vital skill with multiple benefits - from establishing boundaries, prioritizing self-care, maintaining focus on goals, enhancing self-esteem, to fostering honest relationships. Although it might be challenging, especially for those used to saying 'yes', practicing it leads to respectful and authentic communication. Remember, saying 'no' is not a weakness, but a testament of strength and self-awareness.

### SPECIFICALLY IN A FAT LOSS

Saying 'no' is a powerful but often underestimated tool in the weight-loss journey. Beyond nutrition, food provides comfort and pleasure, but it's crucial to acknowledge that not all foods are health-promoting and some contribute to weight gain. Consequently, it's vital to learn to say 'no' to certain foods, whether it's a dessert temptation at a restaurant, a colleague's donut offer, or unhealthy food categories like processed snacks or sugary drinks.

In social situations, saying 'no' is critical where unhealthy food options are prevalent. Despite temptations, keeping health goals front and center is key. It's equally important to establish boundaries with others who might push you towards unhealthy choices. You're not responsible for their feelings or actions, even if standing your ground feels awkward.

The ability to say 'no' can foster a healthier relationship with food, allowing you to control your eating habits and make more conscious, healthier choices. It's not about complete food denial, as many nutritious foods are delicious and can be enjoyed moderately. By rejecting certain foods, you can better appreciate and enjoy the healthy ones.

In short, saying 'no' is a crucial instrument for fat loss and a healthier lifestyle. It helps stay on course with weight-loss goals, cultivates a healthier relationship with food, and aligns choices with health priorities. Saying 'no' is about empowerment, not deprivation, and focuses on your needs rather than others. It's a significant ally in your journey to a healthier lifestyle.

## N for NOBODY

Let me emphasize this vital truth: you are responsible for yourself. While we might wish for a cavalry of teachers, parents, friends, or the government to rescue us, their help isn't guaranteed. The responsibility for your well-being lies squarely on your shoulders, regardless of how much support or love others provide.

Depending on others to solve your problems or make your decisions can lead to disappointment and frustration. It's crucial, therefore, to foster self-reliance, resilience, and advocacy for oneself. Use resources and support when needed, but remember, only you can truly steer your life towards the best it can be.

It's natural to seek help during challenging times. However, heavy reliance on others for well-being may result in feelings of helplessness and disappointment. Self-care involves proactively identifying and addressing our physical, emotional, and mental needs. It's about developing self-awareness, setting boundaries, and making decisions aligned with our values and goals.

This doesn't mean we shouldn't ask for help. Seeking assistance can signify strength, fostering growth and learning. But remember, we bear the ultimate responsibility for our well-being, and we shouldn't rely on others to solve our problems or make our decisions.

Taking charge of our lives leads to empowerment and autonomy. We learn to trust ourselves and our abilities, bolstering self-esteem and resilience. Self-care is not just essential for our well-being, but it can positively influence our relationships and the world around us. In a nutshell, we should lean on others when needed, but never forget, it's on us to look after ourselves.

## N for NUTRITHERAPY

Nutritional therapy, or nutritherapy, is a health and wellness approach that uses food and nutritional supplements to prevent and address various health issues, such as digestive problems and chronic diseases. It aims to correct nutrient deficiencies and imbalances in the body through diet and supplementation, focusing on a balanced diet of whole foods and specific supplements based on individual health needs.

This method can help manage various health concerns including digestive complications, hormonal imbalances, weight issues, and chronic conditions like diabetes and heart disease. For instance, specific nutrients might aid digestive functions or stabilize blood sugar levels, while anti-inflammatory foods and supplements can improve joint health.

A cornerstone of nutritherapy is personalized treatment. A qualified Nutritherapist assesses each individual's health history, lifestyle, and dietary habits to create a tailored treatment plan, which might include identifying food sensitivities, recommending dietary changes, and suggesting specific supplements.

Nutritherapy's guidance comes from evidence-based research, meaning Nutritherapists need to stay updated on the latest nutrition research and understand the interaction between nutrients and the body's healing processes. Nutritherapy can work independently or in combination with other natural therapies like herbal remedies or acupuncture.

The emphasis of nutritherapy extends beyond addressing specific health issues to overall health promotion and disease prevention. By focusing on individual needs and addressing underlying imbalances, nutritherapy uses food and supplements to promote optimal health and wellness effectively.

## N for NUTRITION AND BEHAVIOR

Nutrition and behavior are interconnected and significantly impact fat loss. Different foods influence our energy levels and moods, thus affecting our motivation to engage in fat loss activities. For example, high-carb meals can boost energy, while high-fat ones might lead to lethargy and lower workout enthusiasm.

Nutrients can also affect brain function. Consuming omega-3 fatty acids from sources like fish enhances cognitive function and mood, and antioxidant-rich foods combat oxidative stress, preventing cognitive decline and mood disorders.

Processed foods high in sugar, salt, and unhealthy fats can provoke addictive behaviors and cravings due to the brain's dopamine release. On the other hand, whole foods provide stable energy, curb cravings, and control compulsive eating.

Behavior also affects nutrition. Stress can lead to overeating, and insufficient sleep can disrupt hormones, causing cravings for high-calorie foods. Practicing mindful eating, being aware of hunger and fullness cues, can aid portion control and prevent overeating.

Setting achievable goals and making plans to reach them, like preparing healthy meals, scheduling regular exercise, and incorporating stress management, can boost your success.

In summary, diet influences mood and behavior, and therefore, your fat loss journey. Prioritizing nutrient-rich foods, practicing mindful eating, and goal setting can improve your nutrition and behavior, facilitating your success in losing fat.

# O

## O for ORGANIZATION

Organization is pivotal to maintaining a healthy diet, including effective meal planning, food preparation, and monitoring progress. Planning meals ensures balanced nutrition, aids in avoiding unhealthy food, and controls calorie intake. This promotes health, saves time, and minimizes grocery expenses by reducing shopping trips and food waste.

A methodical approach to food preparation guarantees the availability of healthy meal options, reducing the lure of unhealthy fast food. Organized diet management allows efficient monitoring, using a food journal or an app to keep an eye on nutrient intake, portion sizes, and highlight areas needing improvement. This accountability supports reaching health goals like fat loss.

A clean eating environment is maintained through organization. Regularly tidying the kitchen, pantry, and fridge ensures easy access and visibility to healthy food, discouraging unhealthy eating. It also eliminates clutter and outdated food, thereby reducing stress and poor eating habits.

Furthermore, organization cultivates healthy habits beyond diet, including regular exercise, self-care, and adequate sleep, essential for overall health. These habits decrease stress and promote a positive mindset, further reinforcing healthy eating.

In conclusion, organization is essential for a healthy diet and overall well-being. Although it demands initial discipline, the benefits of this structured approach outweigh the effort, leading to successful achievement of health goals.

## O for OUTRUN A BAD DIET

The phrase "YOU CAN'T OUTRUN A BAD DIET" underscores that no amount of exercise can negate the impacts of poor dietary choices. Our bodies need food for fuel, and loading up on unhealthy, high-calorie, sugar-rich foods can hinder our performance, regardless of our workout routine.

Research points out that diet plays a larger role than exercise in fat loss and overall health. Exercise is essential for maintaining muscle mass, burning energy, and cardiovascular health, but it can't reverse the negative effects of a poor diet. Regular workouts might not yield significant fat loss or health improvements if coupled with a high-calorie, high-fat diet.

A bad diet doesn't just affect weight management—it can also lead to severe health problems such as heart disease, diabetes, and certain cancers, which can't be counteracted solely by regular exercise.

A poor diet usually consists of processed foods, added sugars, unhealthy fats, and refined grains. These foods are calorie-dense but nutrient-poor. On the other hand, a healthy diet includes whole, minimally processed foods like fruits, vegetables, lean proteins, and whole grains, which are nutrient-rich and less calorie-dense.

Though exercise is key to health and fitness, diet plays an even more crucial role in achieving health goals. To improve health and manage weight, it's necessary to make healthy food choices and limit intake of processed, high-calorie foods. In the pursuit of health and fitness goals, we must remember: you can't outrun a bad diet.

## O for OXYGEN

Oxygen is a vital yet often overlooked component of a healthy lifestyle, akin to our diet. It's essential for life and plays a crucial role in health maintenance.

Oxygen primarily helps our cells generate energy, essential for body functions such as digestion, circulation, and respiration.

Insufficient oxygen leads to energy deficits, causing feelings of tiredness and fatigue.

Oxygen is also instrumental in our immune system, assisting in fighting off infections and diseases and fortifying our natural defenses. Moreover, it's crucial for cardiovascular health, regulating blood pressure and supporting proper heart function. Insufficient oxygen can cause issues like high blood pressure and heart failure.

Exercise is one way to boost oxygen levels. During exercise, our deeper breaths intake more oxygen, raising energy levels and improving health. Regular exercise enhances cardiovascular health, thereby improving oxygen levels.

Deep breathing exercises are another method to increase oxygen intake. Slow, deep breaths can not only elevate oxygen levels but also alleviate stress and anxiety, benefiting individuals with respiratory issues or those who struggle with exercise.

Air quality is another critical factor. Air pollution can adversely affect our health and reduce oxygen levels. Improving air quality in homes and workplaces ensures we breathe clean, oxygen-rich air.

In essence, oxygen is as important as a diet for a healthy lifestyle. It's fundamental to several body functions, from energy production to immune and cardiovascular health. Regular exercise, deep breathing exercises, and enhancing air quality can increase our oxygen levels, enhancing overall health and well-being.

By following this link, you will find tools that can help check and increase your oxygen level:

https://www.the10sprotocol.com/s-s-s-b

# P

## P for PAIN

In the pursuit of fat loss, physical and emotional pain often serve as stumbling blocks. But rather than solely being obstacles, they can act as catalysts for progress and personal growth.

Physical discomfort, a common byproduct of intense exercise, can be disheartening at first. However, consistent training can help your body adapt and grow stronger, turning this discomfort into signs of progress.

Emotional pain, often experienced as a struggle against unhealthy food choices, can be intense but fleeting. Making gradual changes in your diet can lessen this struggle and foster healthier eating habits in the long run.

However, it's crucial to see pain as a potential warning sign. Persistent or sharp physical pain during exercise may indicate overexertion or improper form, and ongoing emotional pain could signal that you're pushing too hard or setting unachievable goals. Both require reevaluating and adjusting your approach to ensure a sustainable health regimen.

While pain can act as a motivator, it's vital to balance this with self-compassion and care. Overpushing can lead to burnout, injury, or emotional distress. Prioritizing rest, recovery, and support from loved ones or professionals is key.

In essence, while pain - both physical and emotional - can be daunting in the fat loss journey, it can also prompt change. Consistent effort and incremental lifestyle changes can transform pain into progress. Yet, it's critical to listen to your body and mind, prioritize self-care, and seek support when necessary to maintain a healthy, sustainable approach.

## P for PALATE

Retraining your palate is a pivotal strategy for sustainable dietary improvement. Our tastes are often programmed to crave salty, sweet, and fatty foods, but we can recondition our taste buds to enjoy whole foods, bolstering long-term health.

This palate reeducation starts with minor changes rather than a radical diet revamp. Slowly incorporating more fruits, vegetables, lean proteins, and whole grains can help you appreciate their innate flavors. Experimenting with various cooking techniques and spices is also key. Well-seasoned, healthy foods can be delicious, reducing reliance on unhealthy additions.

Also important is observing your body's response to different foods. Recognizing how foods make you feel—lethargic, bloated, energetic, or content—can inform your food choices. Maintaining a food diary can facilitate this, helping you track progress and identify eating patterns.

Remember, palate reeducation is a gradual process requiring commitment. It's essential to celebrate small wins and continually try new foods and flavors. Besides fostering a healthier diet, this can enhance your enjoyment of eating, ignite a passion for cooking, and boost your appreciation of food's variety and complexity.

In conclusion, re-educating your palate is key to a healthier, sustainable diet. By slowly adding more whole foods and exploring different flavors, you can reset your taste buds to enjoy healthier foods. Over time, you can suppress unhealthy cravings, supporting lifelong health and wellness.

## P for PERSISTENCE

Persistence is the heart of any successful endeavor, especially in dieting and fat loss. The journey towards healthier living can be tough, laden with obstacles and stagnation, but determination pushes you through these challenges.

Staying persistent can mean sticking to a meal plan despite temptations, finding exercise time amidst a hectic day, or tackling a weight-loss plateau without giving up. Persistence is about remaining resolute even when things get difficult.

Having a strong sense of purpose is vital. Knowing why you want to improve your health or lose weight helps you keep your goals in focus. Resilience, too, is key, allowing you to bounce back from setbacks and keep moving forward.

Support is another crucial element of persistence. An exercise buddy for accountability, a friend for moral support, or a professional like a dietitian for advice can be lifesavers during hard times. Patience is also indispensable, as meaningful change takes time and consistent effort.

Celebrating your successes, no matter how small, is essential. Acknowledging progress, be it fat loss, faster running, or simply feeling better, reinforces your motivation and commitment.

In summary, persistence is fundamental to dieting and fat loss success. It involves enduring trials, understanding your motivation, resilience, having support, patience, and celebrating achievements. Armed with these traits, anyone can attain their health goals and foster a healthier lifestyle.

## P for PHOTO

Embarking on a diet can feel daunting, with progress seeming sluggish. A 'before' photo can serve as a powerful motivational tool in this process. It records your starting point and shows how much progress you've made.

Particularly for those targeting fat loss, a pre-diet photo can be insightful. Weighing scales may not fully reflect your progress due to various factors affecting fat loss. However, a photo can vividly display changes in your body composition.

Capture a full-body shot in fitting attire or swimwear to track your transformation. Ensure the photo has good lighting, a plain background, and repeat the same positioning for future photos.

Photos can reveal changes in areas often overlooked when focusing on specific body parts. Regular photos allow you to notice changes across your body and adjust your regimen accordingly.

Remember to take frequent progress photos to monitor your transformation and stay motivated. If progress plateaus, comparing current and previous photos can help spot changes in diet or workout routines.

However, don't solely rely on visual changes for measuring success. While the photos provide a visual log, it's equally important to recognize non-visible improvements like increased energy and overall health.

In summary, 'before' photos are valuable in motivating and tracking progress. They allow you to visualize your journey, celebrate milestones, and, when used regularly, assist in fine-tuning your strategy. Embrace the visible transformations along with the unseen health benefits during your diet journey.

## P for PLAN

Planning is crucial for success, including maintaining a healthy diet. It aids in organization, goal-setting, and motivation, facilitating adherence to dietary goals.

A plan brings structure to your diet, assisting in time management, task prioritization, and effective use of resources. It's especially useful for meal planning, preventing unhealthy eating habits that can emerge when stressed or pressed for time.

A plan also keeps you goal-oriented, helping resist temptations and stay focused despite challenges. This discipline is particularly critical for health goals, such as fat loss.

Furthermore, a plan introduces routine and structure, beneficial for managing food cravings or emotional eating. A stable dietary routine can mitigate these issues, decrease stress and anxiety, and eliminate some uncertainties of maintaining a healthy diet.

Additionally, a plan ensures the intake of essential nutrients and vitamins. Detailed meal planning secures a balanced diet with varied healthy foods, crucial for those with specific dietary needs to maintain optimal health.

Finally, a plan promotes accountability and motivation. A well-defined plan encourages sticking to dietary goals and inspires necessary changes for their realization, fostering a sense of responsibility towards personal health.

In conclusion, planning is vital to a healthy diet, providing structure, guidance, and motivation. Whether your goal is fat loss, health improvement, or a balanced diet, a clear plan can guide you. Invest time in creating a diet plan tailored to you and take a step towards a healthier lifestyle.

## P for PLATEAU

Fat loss plateaus, periods when fat loss pauses despite ongoing efforts, can be disheartening. Understanding why they occur and how to overcome them is vital for sustained fat loss.

Plateaus often happen because as you lose weight, your metabolic rate decreases, meaning you need fewer calories to function. Adjusting caloric intake can keep fat loss on track.

Plateaus can also stem from repetitive diet or exercise routines. Introducing variety keeps your body adaptive and helps prevent this issue.

Stress-induced cortisol spikes can halt fat loss, making stress-management activities like yoga beneficial.

To break a plateau, it's crucial to track and adjust your progress. Documenting food consumption, exercise, and weight changes helps identify required alterations.

Increasing exercise frequency, intensity, or duration can help overcome a plateau. Adding high-intensity interval training (HIIT) or strength exercises can boost metabolism and fat burning.

Dietary modifications, like reducing portion sizes, increasing protein intake, or limiting high-fat, processed foods, can also be effective.

Fat loss isn't a straight path; there will be slow periods. Staying committed to your goals is crucial. Success isn't solely about numbers on a scale. Celebrate non-scale victories like improved energy, mood, and fitting better into your clothes.

To sum up, overcoming a fat loss plateau involves understanding its causes, monitoring progress, increasing physical activity, managing stress, and adjusting your diet. Celebrating all victories, scale or non-scale, is essential for continued motivation towards a healthier lifestyle.

## P for PLAYLIST

Music can be a potent tool in accomplishing diet and fitness goals, offering a wealth of benefits including distraction, mood elevation, enhanced endurance, community building, and the capacity for personalization through playlists.

Using music as a diversion can make workouts more enjoyable and mitigate cravings. Additionally, it has mood-boosting properties, with certain genres prompting brain chemicals like dopamine and serotonin, enhancing motivation.

Interestingly, music can also amplify workout performance. Research indicates it can bolster endurance, making it a valuable asset for those kickstarting fitness routines.

In group fitness scenarios, music can engender a sense of unity, boosting motivation. Crafting personal playlists can further enhance the experience, tailoring the musical journey to your workout intensity or mood.

Despite these benefits, it's essential to remember that musical preference is personal. What motivates one may not resonate with another. Moreover, listening responsibly is crucial; excessive volumes can be detrimental to hearing health.

For music lovers, designated playlists can cater to varied moods or motivation levels, serving as a personalized motivational tool.

In conclusion, music presents an engaging, versatile tool in achieving diet and fitness objectives. With its capacity to distract, uplift mood, improve performance, and foster unity, it's worth experimenting with various genres and playlists to identify what keeps you most motivated.

By following this link, you will find a 3 months FREE Amazon Music that you can cancel at any moment:

https://www.the10sprotocol.com/sport

## P for POISON

Our health is constantly under threat from various environmental pollutants like air and water contamination, harmful substances in our food, and personal care products. Air pollution, laden with harmful particles, can cause respiratory problems, cardiovascular disease, and even cancer. It can also affect our food supply as crops and animals absorb these pollutants.

Water pollution, due to industrial waste and agricultural runoff, can lead to gastrointestinal issues, developmental delays, and cancer. Additionally, toxins from polluted water can contaminate seafood.

Agricultural chemicals and food additives pose serious health risks, such as cancer, reproductive and developmental issues, allergies, and obesity. Certain personal care products carry potential health hazards as well.

Our modern lifestyle choices - stress, insufficient sleep, and unhealthy eating - can amplify these issues by disrupting our body's detoxification process, leading to chronic diseases like autoimmune conditions, allergies, and cancer.

In conclusion, environmental toxins pose significant threats to our health. Mitigating their impact requires reducing exposure, consuming whole foods, using natural products, and supporting our body's detox process through regular exercise, stress management, and sufficient sleep.

You will be able to find everything you need through the following website:

https://www.the10sprotocol.com/detox

## P for POSITIVE THINKING

A positive mindset can significantly influence your fat loss journey, focusing on progress rather than perfection and celebrating small victories. The key lies in self-compassion - being kind to yourself when facing obstacles and remembering that consistency matters more than flawlessness.

View fat loss not as a burden but as a path to improved health and energy. Use visualization to imagine your goals, which can bolster determination. Cultivate gratitude for life's positives, fostering a motivating and satisfying mindset.

Maintaining positivity involves patience, continuous effort, and combating negative thoughts. Though challenging, the benefits include improved mental well-being and self-esteem. Seek support from others - a community or loved ones - to fortify your resolve.

In conclusion, positive thinking is a vital asset in successful fat loss. By emphasizing progress, exercising self-compassion, and showing gratitude, you can enrich your fat loss journey. Positivity, persistence, and support will not only help you reach your goals but also lead to a more fulfilling life.

## P for POTENTIAL

Dietary success is about more than fat loss or physique. It's about unleashing our human potential for a fulfilling life. A healthy diet is essential, but there's more to consider.

The journey starts with defining clear, attainable goals. Understand your reasons for diet changes and your end-goals, like improved health or boosted self-confidence. Break these down into daily achievable steps.

Motivation is crucial. Setbacks are part and parcel of the journey, but maintaining determination and resilience is vital to overcome these challenges.

Establishing wholesome habits - incorporating nutritious foods, regular exercise, adequate sleep, and stress management - is vital. These habits can have far-reaching benefits in all life areas.

Developing self-awareness helps too. Recognize your strengths and areas needing improvement, and be mindful of your thoughts and emotions, particularly when they hinder your progress.

Adopt a growth mindset - believe in your capacity to evolve. View setbacks as opportunities to learn, encouraging curiosity, openness, and the willingness to take risks.

In essence, achieving dietary success involves more than eating right. It requires clear goals, sustained motivation, healthy habits, self-awareness, and a growth mindset. By focusing on these aspects, you can unlock your true potential and lead a fulfilling life.

## P for POWERLESS FEELING

The journey to lose excess body fat can be challenging, particularly when combating both physiological and psychological food cravings. However, with dedicated and consistent changes to your diet, sleep habits, and overall lifestyle, you can gain control over your impulses and steer your health in the desired direction. Achieving your fat loss goals is a realistic expectation, needing perseverance and resilience.

The struggle to overcome long-standing weight issues is complex, involving more than just willpower. Our bodies and minds are intricate systems, and many factors can sway our health and eating habits. With steady and maintainable adjustments, you can shift your body's natural balance towards a healthier state. Even if progress seems slow, every positive step is a stride towards your final goal.

Essentially, it's vital to practice self-compassion. Nobody is perfect, and stumbles are part of any health journey. When you encounter setbacks, avoid self-criticism. Instead, reflect on the cause and how to adapt. Each hurdle is a chance to grow, and every triumph, no matter how minor, deserves celebration.

With determination and commitment to your well-being, you can reshape your relationship with food and your body, leading to enduring fat loss. Keep advancing, stay focused on your objectives, and don't shy away from seeking help when required. You're capable of achieving this!

## P for PRECISION

Hitting dietary targets is a game of precision. It's all about getting the small details right, from tallying calories to controlling portions. Monitoring food intake is crucial; it helps understand caloric consumption, spot eating trends, and allows for necessary modifications.

Portion measurement is essential too. Use tools like food scales and portion control plates to consume accurate amounts, eliminating guesswork that might hamper progress. Precision also extends to food choice - understanding nutrition labels, being aware of portion sizes, and selecting foods that keep us full and energetic.

Exercise isn't exempt from precision. Don't just go through the motions. Ensure correct form and technique, progressively up the intensity, and monitor your progress.

Set detailed, measurable goals and sketch a roadmap to achieve them. These goals could range from losing a specific weight by a certain date or clocking in a set number of daily steps or workout minutes.

Precision boosts accountability. Accurate food and exercise tracking creates a reliable record of our actions, driving results, keeping us motivated, and spotlighting areas for improvement.

Crucially, precision helps avoid an unhealthy fixation on food or exercise. It provides insight into our habits without letting them dominate our lives, promoting a healthy balance and avoiding harmful extremes.

In essence, precision is key for dietary triumph. It enables informed decisions, goal setting, and achieving desired outcomes. Through deliberate actions, you can foster a healthier, more joyful life. Remember, a scientific approach—tracking, experimenting, adjusting—is vital for reaching your fitness goals. With commitment and precision, you can reshape your life.

## P for PROCRASTINATION

"THE COST OF PROCRASTINATION IS THE LIFE YOU COULD HAVE LIVED & THE VERSION OF YOURSELF THAT YOU COULD HAVE BECOME." This sentence is so powerful that you need to print it and put it on your fridge.

Procrastination, a significant obstacle in adhering to a healthy diet, is often driven by feelings of being overwhelmed, unmotivated, or fear of failure. When people are accustomed to unhealthy eating, significant dietary changes can seem daunting. But it's crucial to remember that these changes can be gradual, beginning with simple alterations like adding more fruits and veggies or reducing sugar intake.

Lack of motivation is another challenge. To combat this, set achievable goals and reward yourself for reaching them. Enlisting support from family and friends can boost motivation through accountability and encouragement. Additionally, the fear of failing to stick to a diet plan often induces procrastination. It's essential to understand that occasional mishaps are normal, and the focus should be on the health advantages of a balanced diet.

Procrastination can lead to unhealthy eating habits, weight gain, and health issues. To overcome this, identify and tackle procrastination triggers promptly. Breaking down the intimidating task of a diet overhaul into smaller, feasible steps can help, like replacing unhealthy snacks with healthier ones or reducing portion sizes.

Developing a plan with specific goals, timelines, and meal prep can curb impulsive unhealthy choices. Addressing psychological factors like anxiety or depression, which can fuel procrastination, is also crucial. Consulting a mental health professional can be beneficial in addressing these issues. Understanding the root causes of procrastination, creating effective strategies to counter it, and addressing mental health concerns are critical steps towards a balanced, healthy diet.

By following this link, you will find tools that can help fight your procrastination and increase your productivity:

https://www.the10sprotocol.com/self-discipline

## P for PROGRESS

Progress plays a central role in the success of a diet. It serves as a momentum builder, instilling motivation, and providing a sense of achievement. By setting and attaining small, attainable goals, you create a positive cycle, boosting your drive to overcome challenges and maintain your diet.

Besides this, progress enhances self-confidence. As you reach goals and milestones, you gain mastery over your diet and health, boosting self-esteem and fostering belief in your abilities, which can positively spill over into other aspects of your life.

Monitoring your progress also allows for necessary course corrections. This way, you can promptly spot any deviations from your plan, make the needed adjustments, and ensure you're still on track towards your ultimate goal.

Moreover, recognizing progress nurtures a growth mindset, transforming setbacks into learning opportunities and fostering resilience. Remember, progress isn't always a straight line; there will be highs and lows.

To track your progress effectively, set specific, measurable goals, such as fat loss targets or improving sleep habits. Breaking down larger goals into smaller, manageable steps can simplify tracking progress and enhance motivation.

In essence, monitoring progress, acknowledging achievements, making necessary adjustments, and fostering a growth mindset are vital steps towards enduring health changes. Keep pushing, stay focused on your progress, and you'll be amazed at what you can accomplish.

## P for PROTEIN

Protein, an essential macronutrient found in foods like meats, dairy, beans, and nuts, is indispensable for numerous bodily functions like tissue repair, enzyme production, hormone creation, and immune function support. It's particularly crucial in the diets of athletes and physically active individuals, aiding muscle growth and recovery.

Beyond physical activity, protein contributes significantly to weight management. High-protein diets can diminish appetite, enhance satiety, and reduce calorie intake, aiding fat loss. Additionally, proteins have a high thermic effect, resulting in the body burning more calories and digesting them compared to carbohydrates or fats.

Protein also benefits bone health, maintaining bone density and reducing osteoporosis risk—a significant factor for women prone to bone loss with age. Furthermore, protein positively impacts blood sugar regulation, as its co-consumption with carbohydrates can slow sugar absorption, mitigating blood sugar spikes and crashes.

Not all protein sources offer equal benefits. Red and processed meats, despite being high in protein, can increase heart disease and cancer risk. Hence, lean proteins like poultry, fish, beans, and nuts are recommended. Protein requirements vary based on factors such as age, gender, weight, and physical activity level, with the general rule being at least 1 gram of protein per pound of body weight daily.

However, lack of protein can lead to a range of health issues, from muscle mass loss to weakened immunity, enzyme and hormone production reduction, neurological problems, anemia, poor skin and nail health, and delayed wound healing. Severe deficiency can lead to kwashiorkor, characterized by swollen bellies and thin limbs.

In conclusion, protein is integral to a healthy diet, with a myriad of roles in bodily functions. Consuming sufficient protein from diverse sources supports optimal health and wellness. Balance and moderation in protein intake, prioritizing lean protein sources, are key for maximum health benefits. Ensuring adequate protein intake in our diets is vital for maintaining health and well-being.

By following this link, you will find the best and cleanest protein in the market:

https://www.the10sprotocol.com/supplements

## P for PSYCHOLOGY

Psychology plays a substantial role in shaping our eating habits and food choices, influenced by our thoughts, emotions, and beliefs. Key aspects include emotional eating, where food becomes a stress-coping mechanism, often leading to overeating and unhealthy choices. By identifying emotional triggers, we can better manage these responses and avoid emotional eating.

Habit formation is another critical psychological element. Our unconscious behaviors, influenced by repetition and reinforcement, shape our eating patterns. Strategies like goal setting, progress monitoring, and positive reinforcement can assist in fostering healthier habits.

Our perceptions of food, formed by beliefs and attitudes, significantly impact our choices. Understanding these beliefs, and avoiding labels like "good" or "bad" foods, can encourage a healthier food relationship. Additionally, recognizing willpower's finite nature can help devise strategies to conserve it, making healthier choices easier.

Overcoming setbacks in changing eating habits can be aided by psychological strategies such as self-monitoring, social support, and mindfulness. Moreover, understanding social and cultural influences on our eating habits can empower informed food choices and assist in reaching health goals.

In sum, psychology provides invaluable insights into eating habits and behaviors. By leveraging psychological strategies, we can better navigate emotional eating, habit formation, and other challenges, empowering us to achieve our health goals.

## P for FOOD PYRAMID

The once-popular food pyramid is being reconsidered for its potential negative impacts on diets. Its broad approach doesn't account for individual differences like age, gender, physical activity, or health conditions, potentially causing imbalances in food consumption.

For example, the pyramid's emphasis on grains and carbohydrates could contribute to blood sugar irregularities, insulin resistance, and weight gain in some individuals. Its dairy recommendations might be unsuitable for those with lactose intolerance or allergies.

The pyramid's preference for carbohydrates over healthy fats and proteins may contradict current nutrition science, which indicates that high-carb diets might increase the risk of chronic diseases like diabetes and heart disease.

Moreover, the pyramid could instill damaging cultural attitudes towards food, categorizing foods as "good" or "bad," potentially promoting guilt, shame, and disordered eating. There's also concern that the pyramid may be more influenced by commercial interests and political agendas than scientific evidence, possibly over-promoting certain foods due to industry pressures.

In summary, while the food pyramid has historically promoted healthy eating, its general approach, potential cultural biases, and possible deviation from current nutritional science might negatively influence our diets. A tailored approach to nutrition, guided by professionals, can better ensure health needs are met.

## Q for QUALITY vs QUANTITY

### IN FOOD

A balanced diet isn't just about quantity, but also the quality of food consumed. The impact of 100 calories from nutrient-dense vegetables differs significantly from the same amount from a sugar-loaded soda. High-quality foods, rich in essential nutrients, are satisfying and decrease the inclination to snack on unhealthy items.

Diets abundant in processed foods, sugar, and unhealthy fats can lead to health issues like obesity, diabetes, and heart disease. Conversely, diets centered around unprocessed foods reduce these risks, fostering overall health.

Whole foods, such as fresh fruits, vegetables, whole grains, lean proteins, and healthy fats, contribute to a high-quality diet. When picking packaged foods, look for options with whole food ingredients and minimal additives.

However, even with high-quality foods, portion control is essential, as overeating can occur. Tools like measuring cups or food scales can assist in maintaining correct portion sizes. Additionally, mindful eating—eating slowly and without distractions—helps recognize hunger and fullness cues, thus minimizing overeating.

In summary, focusing on food quality is critical for a healthy diet. Emphasizing unprocessed, whole foods and managing portion sizes not only provides essential nutrients but also reduces chronic disease risks. Healthy eating hinges on what you eat, not merely how much.

## IN WORKOUT

In pursuit of fitness, the quality of your workout, along with a balanced diet, holds as much significance as the quantity of exercise you perform. Prioritizing quality not only boosts fitness results but also guards against injuries that could halt your progress, often caused by rushing or compromising form for the sake of more reps.

By focusing on correct form and technique, your workouts become more efficient, leading to increased strength, better endurance, and enhanced calorie burn. Such quality-oriented workouts yield mental health benefits too, offering stress relief and mood elevation, particularly when you choose exercises that you enjoy and feel comfortable with.

Contrary to popular belief, quality workouts don't necessarily mean longer or more intense routines. They emphasize the proper execution of exercises without risking injury or fatigue, fostering consistency.

A crucial aspect of quality workouts is that they support long-term lifestyle changes. They encourage you to prioritize personal needs over societal expectations, paving the way for a more intuitive approach to exercise and diet.

In a nutshell, while workout quantity has its place, quality exercises combined with a healthy diet are crucial for sustainable success. Focusing on form and technique over reps or weight not only helps avoid injuries and enhances results but also reduces stress and nurtures a more intuitive approach to fitness, leading to a healthier, long-term lifestyle.

# R

## R for REALITY CHECK

Realistic expectations and regular reality checks are essential in your diet and fat loss journey. Setting goals too high can lead to disappointment and giving up, so it's important to understand that fat loss isn't a straight path and hurdles are bound to occur.

Frequent reality checks encourage honesty about your lifestyle habits. It may reveal hard truths like overeating or lack of exercise, but it also gives a clear idea about where you need to improve.

Regular reality checks also help in setting achievable goals. Losing weight healthily is a slow process, usually around 1-2 pounds per week, so setting realistic targets can guide you towards success without risking failure.

Reality checks also help maintain motivation and focus on your goals. They remind you of your wins and losses, even if progress is not always linear.

Reality checks help you remember the bigger picture: the long-term benefits of a healthier lifestyle, including improved health, energy, and self-confidence. This perspective keeps you committed and positive, even when facing setbacks.

Finally, reality checks can prevent burnout. Acknowledging both your achievements and obstacles along the way helps to keep a balanced perspective and prevents feeling overwhelmed.

In conclusion, reality checks are vital in dieting and fat loss plans. They provide grounding, aid in setting realistic goals, maintain motivation, and prevent burnout. By being truthful with yourself and acknowledging your progress and setbacks, you can achieve lasting success and lead a healthier lifestyle.

## R for REBELLION

Living a healthy lifestyle means adopting a proactive attitude towards our health and challenging defeatist mindsets that view unhealthy states as unchangeable. Accepting an unhealthy lifestyle can breed complacency and future health issues.

Remember, your current health state isn't permanent. There are always ways to improve, such as dietary changes, increased exercise, or professional health advice.

Also, avoid blaming yourself for unhealthy habits. Our environment plays a significant role in influencing our health choices. Instead, focus on small lifestyle changes, like reducing sugar, eating more fruits and vegetables, or walking daily. These incremental changes can considerably improve health over time.

Seek support from friends, family, or professionals when needed. Lifestyle changes can be daunting, and having a supportive network can be invaluable.

Lastly, see your health as a worthwhile investment. Don't shy away from lifestyle changes out of fear of cost or time. Investing in your health now can prevent future costs tied to poor health, such as large medical bills and lost workdays. Plus, this investment can lead to a happier, healthier, and potentially longer life.

In conclusion, it's essential to resist viewing an unhealthy state as unchangeable. Emphasize gradual lifestyle changes, seek support when necessary, and recognize your health as a worthwhile investment. With determination, a healthier life is within reach.

## R for REBORN

Starting a diet can feel like a rebirth, signaling a transformative shift away from old habits towards healthier ones. This journey, though challenging, can bring newfound energy, focus, and purpose.

Dieting necessitates an overhaul of eating habits, replacing processed, high-calorie foods with nutrient-dense alternatives like fruits, vegetables, and lean proteins. This process can deepen appreciation for healthy eating's power.

Accompanying dietary changes, a renewed commitment to exercise arises, offering various health benefits like fat loss, boosted energy levels, and improved mood. These positive impacts can make one feel reborn into a healthier self.

Dieting also sparks a mindset shift. Food transforms from a source of comfort or stress relief to a means of fueling the body. This shift brings mindfulness to eating habits, promoting a sense of empowerment and control.

Furthermore, dieting can help reconnect the mind and body, especially for those feeling a disconnect due to weight issues. This reconnection fosters overall health and well-being.

Finally, dieting provides an opportunity for self-discovery, breaking free from negative self-perceptions and fostering self-worth as progress becomes apparent.

In conclusion, dieting can be a transformative, almost rebirth-like experience. Through dietary changes, exercise commitment, and mindset shift, individuals can gain energy, purpose, and empowerment. Embracing this journey allows for self-discovery and significant life changes.

## R for RECOVERY

Achieving a healthy lifestyle requires not only balanced eating and regular exercise but also a commitment to recovery. This important component, often overlooked, includes relaxation and rejuvenation of both the body and mind.

Sleep is vital to recovery, allowing the body to undergo essential physical and mental repair processes. It also facilitates tissue regeneration, immune system strengthening, cognitive function enhancement, and helps manage appetite and metabolism.

Recovery also encompasses post-workout activities such as stretching, massages, and foam rolling. Regular rest days or active recovery days can help prevent injuries and promote healing.

It's crucial to remember recovery extends beyond physical rest to include mental and emotional recuperation. Persistent stress over diet and exercise can harm health and fat loss efforts. Techniques like meditation, deep breathing, or quiet introspection, along with activities such as outdoor walks or yoga, can help alleviate stress.

Recovery also involves properly fueling your body with nutrient-dense foods to aid repair and regeneration, and staying hydrated to support optimal body functions and toxin elimination.

In conclusion, incorporating recovery into your health regimen can greatly enhance progress and sustainability. Prioritizing rest and relaxation supports not just injury prevention and stress reduction, but also overall well-being. Hence, it's essential to include recovery in your health plan.

## R for REGENERATION

Regeneration, the body's natural healing and restoration process, is crucial for health and greatly influenced by our lifestyle choices, particularly diet. Consuming anti-inflammatory and nutrient-rich foods can enhance our body's regenerative abilities.

Regenerative diets, abundant in fruits, vegetables, whole grains, and healthy fats, can reduce inflammation, a common cause of many chronic diseases, while promoting overall healing. Such diets support a healthy digestive system, breaking down food into absorbable nutrients and aiding waste elimination. High-fiber foods can also offset the negative impacts of processed or fried foods.

Our skin, hair, and nails, which are constantly regenerating, benefit from a diet rich in essential vitamins and minerals. Similarly, to counteract natural age-related deterioration of muscles and bones, a diet high in protein, calcium, and vitamin D is recommended.

To optimize regeneration, balance your diet with whole grains, fruits, vegetables, lean proteins, and healthy fats, limit processed foods, and stay hydrated. Tune into your body's hunger and fullness signals, and observe how different foods affect you. Pairing a regenerative diet with regular physical activity boosts circulation and supports muscle and bone health, emphasizing the importance of regeneration in maintaining overall health.

## R for REGRETS

Dieting can stir up various emotions, often prompting regrets such as wishing you'd started earlier, having quit too soon, or feeling isolated in your efforts. Instead of lingering on these regrets, use them as motivation to kickstart your journey, commit consistently, and seek companionship for support and accountability.

Be wary of trendy diets offering quick fixes; they're typically unsustainable and can pose health risks. Choose a balanced, long-term diet with nutrient-rich foods and regular exercise instead. Remember, skipping meals isn't the solution; it slows metabolism, drains energy, and triggers overeating. Opt for balanced, regular meals and snacks. It's fine to indulge occasionally, just be sure to return to healthier choices afterward.

Steer clear of negative self-talk and guilt; they'll only obstruct your progress. Celebrate minor achievements and foster a positive outlook. In a nutshell, regard your dieting regrets as lessons, avoid common diet pitfalls, and stick to a sustainable routine. There's no perfect time to start other than now. Don't allow past regrets to hinder your path towards your goals.

## R for RELAPSE

Experiencing a dieting relapse, or slipping back into old, unhealthy habits, is quite common. Rather than viewing this as a defeat, think of it as a chance for personal growth. Relapses are often prompted by stress, emotional unrest, or feelings of food deprivation, leading to negative emotions and unhealthy patterns.

Confronting a relapse directly, rather than dismissing it, enables you to shift focus from failure to understanding your triggers and creating strategies to bypass them next time. Remember, a relapse doesn't erase past progress. Gained weight isn't everlasting, and with positivity and strategy, you can reestablish your healthful journey.

Avoid future relapses by identifying triggers, implementing coping mechanisms, setting realistic goals, and having a supportive network. Know your triggers and create healthy responses, such as exercise or talking with a friend. By breaking down your overall goal into manageable steps and celebrating each victory, you prevent feeling overwhelmed.

Involving friends, family, or support groups can promote healthier habits. If a relapse becomes overwhelming, professional help can be invaluable. In essence, relapses are normal, and should be seen as learning opportunities rather than failures.

## R for RELAXING

Relaxation holds a critical role in dieting, akin to the significance of food intake and exercise. It contributes to stress reduction, as chronic stress can provoke weight gain, disturbed sleep, and unhealthy eating. Using relaxation techniques such as meditation, deep breathing, and yoga can mitigate stress levels.

Additionally, these techniques can also improve sleep quality, a key factor for fat loss and overall health. Relaxation helps control food cravings, which are often driven by the stress hormone cortisol. It also promotes healthier digestion by countering the stress-induced "fight or flight" response that can cause digestive issues.

Moreover, relaxation aids in mood enhancement, mitigating symptoms of depression and anxiety and encouraging healthier choices. To incorporate relaxation into your diet routine, set aside dedicated time for it, choose a technique that suits you, and practice consistently. Variety in relaxation methods can keep it enjoyable and prevent monotony.

Ultimately, relaxation shouldn't feel like a task, but rather an enjoyable activity. In conclusion, relaxation is an essential aspect of dieting, helping to alleviate stress, improve sleep, control cravings, enhance digestion, and boost mood, all contributing to your overall health journey.

## R for REQUESTING HELP

Starting a diet might be intimidating, but remember, you're not alone. Securing support from a friend, relative, or professional can greatly simplify your journey to healthier habits. Such assistance offers accountability, meaning someone monitors your progress and motivates you, preventing you from straying off your diet plan. This guidance ensures a smoother and more enjoyable path towards your goals.

In times of uncertainty regarding realistic targets or dieting choices, a knowledgeable ally can help you craft a feasible plan, keeping you concentrated and reminding you of your initial motivations.

Experts can help you avoid common dieting blunders like under or overeating, and guide you on optimal food choices and timings. Participating in a community fosters a sense of camaraderie and connection to others on similar journeys, pushing you to succeed not only for yourself but for your team.

Lastly, having a support system allows for the development of lasting healthy habits, as you learn new strategies and stay motivated and accountable even amidst life's challenges.

In essence, seeking help when dieting comes with multiple advantages, including accountability, better goal-setting, mistake-avoidance, community-building, and sustainable healthy habits creation. If you're thinking of dieting, consider seeking help - it might just be the key to your success.

## R for RESET

Attaining fat loss and a healthier lifestyle often requires a "reset" of habits, such as a short fast or a cleansing diet. This break in routine helps disrupt old habits, eliminate toxins, and promote healthier cravings.

Common forms of reset include a sugar detox, often lasting one to four weeks, which can be challenging due to sugar's addictive nature, but leads to reduced inflammation, improved insulin sensitivity, and curbed sweet cravings.

Another option is a whole food cleanse, focusing on nutrient-rich whole foods, helping with fat loss and providing essential nutrients. Some might find it beneficial to remove foods they're intolerant to, which lets the body heal and reduces inflammation.

Alternatively, a more sustainable reset can simply involve focusing on a balanced diet with fruits, vegetables, lean proteins, and healthy fats. Resets help break unhealthy habits that block fat loss progress, but they aren't quick fixes, rather, they're tools for kickstarting long-term changes.

In conclusion, a reset, be it sugar detox, whole foods cleanse, or a balanced diet, can help push significant changes towards your fat loss goals.

## R for ROUTINE

Establishing a routine is a potent tool for sustaining a healthy diet. It fosters beneficial habits, reduces stress, and introduces structure and regularity to our day-to-day lives.

Routines can make healthy choices feel automatic and effortless. Adhering to an eating schedule can deter meal skipping or unhealthy snacking, while promoting metabolic and digestive functions, key for weight management.

Routines also help ease stress and anxiety by allowing us to efficiently manage our time and tasks, reducing decision fatigue and freeing up mental capacity for other essential tasks. Moreover, they bolster accountability and motivation.

A well-planned meal and exercise routine increase our chances of achieving goals, a boon for those who struggle with self-discipline or are easily derailed by unforeseen circumstances or temptations. They also promote mindful eating; planning meals ahead ensures we get necessary nutrients and enables us to make healthier choices rather than succumbing to convenience or cravings.

Importantly, routines don't equate to a lack of variety or spontaneity. You can build a flexible routine that allows for some food and meal-time variations while keeping healthy habits.

In essence, dietary routines bring numerous benefits like better physical and mental health, increased accountability, and a mindful food approach. Though establishing a routine takes time and effort, its long-term benefits make it a worthy investment for health and wellness goals.

# S

## S for SLEEP

I have written a book called the 10S PROTOCOL where I emphasize 10 points in particular that are crucial for an effective fat loss. SLEEP is one of the 10S.

Indeed, in the bustling world of fat loss strategies, one vital element often takes a back seat: sleep. Yet, if you're on a mission to shed those stubborn pounds, understanding the profound influence of sleep on your body is a game-changer.

The connection between sleep and fat loss isn't some far-fetched notion; it's grounded in science and profoundly impacts your journey toward a healthier you. Let's delve deeper into the importance of sleep in the context of losing fat.

**Metabolism in Repose**: While you're peacefully slumbering, your body is hard at work, repairing and rejuvenating itself. This restorative process has a direct impact on your metabolism. During deep sleep, metabolic functions are optimized, ensuring efficient calorie expenditure even at rest. Inadequate sleep disrupts this delicate balance, leading to a sluggish metabolism and reduced fat-burning potential.

**Hormones and Hunger**: Sleep is the master regulator of your hormones, especially leptin and ghrelin. Leptin signals fullness, while ghrelin triggers hunger. A lack of sleep throws this finely tuned system into disarray, causing an increase in ghrelin levels and a decrease in leptin. The result? Heightened cravings for calorie-dense, sugary foods, making it challenging to resist the siren call of unhealthy snacks.

**Energy for Exercise**: Fat loss isn't just about what you eat; it's also about how active you are. Physical activity is a vital component of any weight loss plan. However, without adequate sleep, you're likely to feel fatigued and lacking in energy. This can be a significant obstacle to maintaining a consistent exercise routine, as your motivation wanes and your workout performance suffers.

**Stress Management**: Sleep plays a pivotal role in stress management. A well-rested body is better equipped to handle daily stressors. In contrast, chronic stress can lead to overeating and poor food choices. Moreover, stress triggers the release of cortisol, a hormone associated with fat storage, especially around the abdominal area. Adequate sleep acts as a natural stress-reducer, helping you manage stress and curb cortisol levels.

**Consistency is Key**: Establishing a regular sleep schedule helps regulate your body's internal clock, or circadian rhythm. This regularity extends to your eating habits, promoting healthier food choices. It's easier to resist late-night snacking when you're well-rested and have a consistent sleep routine.

**Muscle Recovery**: When you're aiming to lose fat, preserving lean muscle mass is essential. Quality sleep is crucial for muscle recovery and repair. During deep sleep phases, growth hormone is released, which aids in muscle repair and growth. Inadequate sleep disrupts this process, potentially leading to muscle loss instead of fat loss.

**The Brain-Sleep Connection**: Sleep deprivation affects your cognitive function and decision-making abilities. When you're tired, you're more likely to make impulsive, unhealthy food choices. This can sabotage your fat loss efforts by causing you to reach for comfort foods rather than nutritious options.

In summary, sleep isn't a luxury; it's a fundamental component of any effective fat loss plan. To optimize your body's fat-burning potential, aim for 7-9 hours of quality sleep each night. Prioritizing sleep alongside a balanced diet and regular exercise will help you achieve your fat loss goals more effectively and sustainably.

In the grand tapestry of weight loss, sleep is a thread that ties everything together. It affects your metabolism, your hormones, your energy levels, your stress management, your consistency, your muscle recovery, and even your decision-making. So, if you're looking to unlock the full potential of your fat loss journey, don't underestimate the power of a good night's sleep—it might just be the key to your success.

By following the link below, you will discover more about the TOOLS that can help improve your SLEEP: https://www.the10sprotocol.com/sleep

## S for SATAN'S FOOD vs SUPERFOOD

I have written a book called the 10S PROTOCOL where I emphasize 10 points in particular that are crucial for an effective fat loss. Avoiding Junk Food and choosing instead Superfood is one of the 10S.

Indeed, in the never-ending struggle to shed those stubborn pounds, our diet plays a pivotal role. The choices we make when it comes to food can either be the wind beneath our wings or the anchor that drags us down. In this epic battle of good versus evil, it's the clash between junk food and superfoods that takes center stage. Let's delve into the importance of these dietary choices in the quest to lose fat.

**Junk Food: The Tempting Culprit**

Junk food, with its tantalizing aroma and addictive flavors, often beckons like a siren to the weary traveler on the path to fat loss. Burgers, fries, sugary sodas, and processed snacks are among its infamous arsenal. These foods are packed with empty calories, sugar, unhealthy fats, and an array of artificial additives. While they may momentarily satisfy our cravings, they come at a hefty cost.

One of the primary drawbacks of junk food is its calorie density. Consuming these foods typically results in a calorie surplus, which leads to fat gain. Moreover, the high sugar content can wreak havoc on our blood sugar levels, causing energy crashes and intensifying cravings. The trans fats found in many junk foods contribute to inflammation and hinder fat loss by interfering with insulin sensitivity.

## Superfoods: Nature's Fat Loss Allies

On the flip side, we have the superheroes of the culinary world – superfoods. These nutrient-packed powerhouses offer a wealth of benefits to those seeking to lose fat. Think of berries, leafy greens, lean proteins, nuts, seeds, and whole grains. These foods are rich in vitamins, minerals, antioxidants, and fiber, making them essential tools in the battle against fat.

The secret weapon of superfoods is their ability to keep you full and satisfied, thanks to their high fiber content. Fiber slows down digestion, helping to regulate blood sugar levels and prevent energy crashes. This, in turn, reduces those nagging cravings for sugary, calorie-laden junk.

Moreover, the vitamins and minerals in superfoods play a pivotal role in metabolic processes. For example, B vitamins help convert food into energy, while magnesium is essential for regulating insulin sensitivity. These nutrients ensure that your body functions optimally, promoting efficient fat loss.

## The Battle Plan: Striking a Balance

In the quest to lose fat, the importance of the junk food versus superfood showdown cannot be overstated. While it may be tempting to eliminate junk food entirely, it's often an unrealistic approach in the long run. Moderation is the key. Instead of succumbing to the allure of junk food, treat it as an occasional indulgence rather than a daily staple.

A balanced diet that incorporates superfoods is the winning strategy. A plate filled with colorful vegetables, lean protein, and whole grains not only nourishes your body but also keeps you on track in your fat loss journey. Superfoods help you maintain a calorie deficit, which is the cornerstone of weight loss, without leaving you feeling deprived.

## Conclusion: The Verdict

In the battle of the bulge, junk food and superfoods are formidable adversaries, each with its own strengths and weaknesses. Junk food may be a tantalizing foe, but its empty calories and detrimental effects on blood sugar levels make it a perilous choice for those seeking fat loss. Superfoods, on the other hand, are the valiant heroes, offering a bounty of nutrients, fiber, and satiety that aid in shedding those unwanted pounds.

To win the war on fat, it's crucial to strike a balance. Embrace superfoods as your allies, and let junk food be an occasional treat rather than a daily opponent. In this way, you can harness the power of nutrition to achieve your fat loss goals, ultimately emerging victorious in the battle of junk food versus superfoods.

By following the link below, you will discover more about the TOOLS that can help improve your relation with food, count the calories etc.: https://www.the10sprotocol.com/satans-food-vs-superfood

## S for SELF-DISCIPLINE

I have written a book called the 10S PROTOCOL where I emphasize 10 points in particular that are crucial for an effective fat loss. SELF-DISCIPLINE is one of the 10S.

Indeed, in the quest to shed excess body fat and achieve a healthier, leaner physique, one fundamental element stands out as an unwavering pillar of success: self-discipline. In a world brimming with temptations and distractions, the ability to exercise self-control and make mindful choices about our dietary habits and lifestyle plays a pivotal role in our journey towards effective and sustainable fat loss.

### Understanding Self-Discipline

Before diving into the importance of self-discipline in losing fat, it's crucial to grasp what self-discipline truly means. Self-discipline is not about punishment or deprivation; it's about making conscious decisions that align with your long-term goals, even when faced with immediate gratification or convenience.

### The Dietary Dilemma

When it comes to losing fat, your dietary choices carry immense weight. It's all too easy to succumb to the allure of high-calorie, low-nutrition foods that provide momentary pleasure but hinder your progress. This is where self-discipline becomes your most potent weapon.

Self-discipline empowers you to resist the temptation of that sugary dessert, the allure of greasy fast food, and the allure of late-night snacking. It enables you to choose whole, nutrient-dense foods that nourish your body and support your fat loss goals. By consistently making these choices, you create a caloric deficit, which is the foundation of weight loss.

**Consistency is Key**

One of the greatest strengths of self-discipline is its ability to foster consistency. Successful fat loss is not about extreme diets or intense bursts of exercise followed by periods of neglect. It's about maintaining a steady, sustainable approach over time. Self-discipline helps you adhere to your chosen diet and exercise plan day in and day out, ensuring that you stay on track toward your goals.

**Resisting Emotional Eating**

Emotions often play a significant role in our eating habits. Stress, sadness, boredom, and celebration can trigger unhealthy eating patterns. Self-discipline provides you with the tools to recognize these emotional triggers and make choices that serve your long-term well-being rather than offering temporary solace.

**The Role of Habits**

Self-discipline also plays a crucial role in habit formation. Establishing healthy routines and rituals, such as meal prepping, regular exercise, and consistent sleep patterns, requires discipline. Once these habits become ingrained, they no longer feel like a struggle but rather a natural part of your daily life, making fat loss more sustainable in the long run.

**Overcoming Plateaus**

The journey to fat loss is rarely a linear progression. There will be plateaus and setbacks along the way. This is where self-discipline truly shines. When faced with a plateau, self-discipline encourages you to stay committed to your goals, even when progress seems slow or non-existent. It prevents you from giving in to frustration and reverting to unhealthy habits.

**Celebrating Small Wins**

Self-discipline doesn't mean denying yourself all pleasures. It's about making informed choices. It also means celebrating your victories, no matter how small they may seem. Recognizing and rewarding yourself for your progress reinforces the importance of your goals and motivates you to keep going.

**In Conclusion**

In the realm of fat loss, self-discipline is the cornerstone of success. It empowers you to make mindful choices about your diet, exercise, and lifestyle, ultimately leading to sustainable progress. While self-discipline may require effort and practice, the rewards it brings in terms of improved health, self-confidence, and a leaner body are more than worth the investment. So, embrace the power of self-discipline, and let it be your guiding force on the path to achieving your fat loss goals. Remember, it's not about perfection, but progress, and self-discipline will be your steadfast companion on this transformative journey.

You can find its entire courses by following the link below:

https://bit.ly/10SSELFDISCIPLINE

https://www.the10sprotocol.com/self-discipline

## S for SKIN

I have written a book called the 10S PROTOCOL where I emphasize 10 points in particular that are crucial for an effective fat loss. SKIN is one of the 10S.

When embarking on the path to fat loss, we often focus on the numbers on the scale or the inches around our waist. However, there's another crucial aspect of our journey that deserves attention: our skin. The health and condition of your skin are intimately linked to your efforts to shed excess fat. Let's explore why skin health is an essential component of your fat loss journey.

**Elasticity and Tone:**

As you lose fat, your skin can be affected by changes in its elasticity and tone. When you carry excess weight for an extended period, your skin stretches to accommodate the additional fat. While losing fat is a commendable goal, it can sometimes lead to loose or sagging skin. Proper nutrition and hydration play a vital role in maintaining skin elasticity and tone during your fat loss journey.

**Preventing Stretch Marks:**

Rapid weight loss or significant fluctuations in weight can lead to stretch marks. These are a result of the skin's collagen and elastin fibers breaking down due to stretching. While genetics can influence your likelihood of developing stretch marks, keeping your skin well-hydrated and nourished with a balanced diet can help minimize their appearance.

**Skin Health and Glow:**

The foods you consume during your fat loss journey can impact the overall health and appearance of your skin. A diet rich in antioxidants, vitamins, and minerals can promote skin health by protecting it from oxidative damage and promoting collagen production. Incorporating foods like fruits, vegetables, and lean proteins can contribute to a radiant complexion.

**Hydration Matters:**

Proper hydration is not only crucial for overall health but also for maintaining skin health. Dehydrated skin can appear dull and less elastic. Drinking an adequate amount of water helps your skin stay hydrated and plump, which can be particularly important when you're actively losing fat.

**Confidence Boost:**

The condition of your skin can have a significant impact on your self-esteem and body confidence. Taking care of your skin as you work towards your fat loss goals can help you feel more comfortable and confident in your own skin, even as your body undergoes changes.

**Avoiding Skin Irritations:**

As you become more active and engage in exercise routines, proper skincare becomes even more critical. Sweating during workouts can lead to skin issues like acne or rashes. Maintaining good hygiene and adopting a skincare routine that suits your skin type can help prevent these irritations.

In conclusion, the importance of skin health in your fat loss journey cannot be overstated. Your skin is a reflection of your overall health and well-being, and it can be profoundly affected by the choices you make during your fat loss efforts. To achieve the best results, focus not only on the numbers but also on nourishing and caring for your skin. By prioritizing skin health, you'll not only look better but also feel more confident and comfortable as you work towards your fat loss goals.

By following the link below, you will discover more about the TOOLS that can help improve your SKIN :

https://www.the10sprotocol.com/skin

## S for SNOWBALL EFFECT

The "snowball effect" is a concept used to describe the progressive benefits gained from persistent, positive alterations to one's lifestyle, especially in terms of fat loss. It's like a snowball rolling down a hill, gathering more snow and momentum as it goes. As you start shedding weight, your body becomes more adept at calorie burning. Simple changes, like daily exercise, can create a significant ripple effect on your overall calorie consumption. Over time, as the fat loss process continues, your metabolism adjusts, becoming more efficient at fat-burning, thus facilitating quicker fat loss while boosting energy and motivation levels.

This effect also instigates encouraging feedback loops. For instance, witnessing noticeable progress like a lower number on the scale or a decrease in body fat percentage inspires you to stick to your healthy habits, thereby further fueling positive outcomes.

However, the flip side is that reverting to unhealthy behaviors can hinder this momentum, highlighting the importance of sustained commitment to your goals.

The key is to start small, making manageable changes that gradually build momentum. Once one change becomes habitual, introduce another, consistently working towards a healthier lifestyle. Maintaining a positive mindset and being adaptable is crucial. Moreover, remember that fat loss is a highly individual process, so you should find a plan that suits you, possibly with professional guidance. In essence, the snowball effect, when properly harnessed, can significantly aid sustainable fat loss, promoting increased motivation, energy, and success through small, consistent changes over time.

## S for SPORT

I have written a book called the 10S PROTOCOL where I emphasize 10 points in particular that are crucial for an effective fat loss. SPORT is one of the 10S.

In the pursuit of a healthier and leaner physique, the incorporation of sports or physical activities takes center stage. It's not merely about shedding pounds; it's about building a strong and sustainable foundation for fat loss. Let's delve into the profound importance of sports in your journey towards losing fat.

**Maximizing Calorie Burn:**

At its core, fat loss boils down to creating a calorie deficit, where you burn more calories than you consume. Sports are a dynamic way to torch calories effectively. Whether it's swimming, running, cycling, or team sports like soccer or basketball, engaging in physical activities elevates your heart rate and ramps up your metabolism, leading to increased calorie expenditure. This calorie burn persists even after your workout is over, a phenomenon known as the "afterburn effect."

**Preserving Lean Muscle Mass:**

One of the pitfalls of traditional weight loss approaches, such as crash diets, is that they often lead to muscle loss along with fat loss. Sports, on the other hand, help you preserve lean muscle mass. Activities that involve resistance, like weightlifting or bodyweight exercises, are particularly effective in maintaining and even building muscle. More muscle equates to a higher resting metabolic rate, meaning you burn more calories at rest.

### Mental Well-being and Motivation:

The mental aspect of fat loss is often underestimated. The discipline and dedication required to engage in sports can spill over into other areas of your life, including your dietary choices. Sports can serve as a potent motivator, boosting your commitment to your fat loss goals. Moreover, physical activity triggers the release of endorphins, which can significantly improve your mood and reduce stress, making it easier to stick to a healthy eating plan.

### Building a Stronger, More Resilient Body:

Fat loss isn't just about the numbers on the scale; it's about improving your overall health and well-being. Engaging in sports helps build a stronger, more resilient body. It enhances cardiovascular health, increases bone density, and improves flexibility and balance. This holistic approach to fitness ensures that you're not just losing fat but also becoming a healthier version of yourself.

### Enhancing Metabolic Efficiency:

Sports have a transformative effect on your metabolism. Regular physical activity can enhance insulin sensitivity, which means your body becomes more efficient at utilizing glucose for energy. This can be particularly beneficial for individuals dealing with insulin resistance or metabolic syndrome, conditions often associated with excess body fat.

### Sustainable Lifestyle Change:

Many diets and weight loss programs are temporary fixes that fail to address the long-term sustainability of fat loss. Sports, on the other hand, offer a pathway to a sustainable lifestyle change. They provide a sense of purpose and enjoyment that goes beyond the goal of losing fat. When you find joy in physical activity, you're more likely to stick with it over the long haul.

## Social Support and Accountability:

Participating in sports often involves a community or team aspect. This social support can be a game-changer in your fat loss journey. Having workout buddies or teammates can provide accountability, encouragement, and motivation, making it easier to stay committed to your goals.

## Learning About Your Body:

Engaging in sports allows you to develop a deeper understanding of your body's capabilities and limitations. You'll become attuned to how different activities affect your energy levels, appetite, and recovery. This self-awareness empowers you to make informed choices that support your fat loss goals.

## Conclusion: The Power of Sports in Fat Loss

In the journey to lose fat, sports aren't just a means to an end; they are an integral part of the process. Beyond the physical benefits, sports offer a holistic approach to health and well-being, encompassing mental and emotional aspects as well. Whether you're a seasoned athlete or a novice, incorporating sports into your fat loss strategy can transform your body and your life, setting you on a path towards lasting success. So, lace up your sneakers, grab your racket, or dive into the pool, because the world of sports is waiting to propel you towards a leaner, healthier you.

By following the link below, you will discover more about the TOOLS that can help improve your practice of SPORT : https://www.the10sprotocol.com/sport

## S for S.S.S.B

I have written a book called the 10S PROTOCOL where I emphasize 10 points in particular that are crucial for an effective fat loss. Stop Suffocating Start Breathing is one of the 10S.

In the pursuit of fat loss, we often become consumed by calorie counts, workout routines, and dietary restrictions. However, there's an integral aspect of the process that's often overlooked and underestimated: breathing. Yes, something as simple and innate as breathing plays a profound role in your journey to shed unwanted fat. Let's delve into the importance of conscious breathing and its impact on your fat loss goals.

**Oxygenating Fat Cells:**

The process of fat metabolism relies on oxygen. When you breathe deeply and efficiently, you ensure that your body has an ample supply of oxygen. This is vital because oxygen helps break down fat molecules into smaller components that can be used for energy. Without adequate oxygen, the fat-burning process becomes less efficient.

**Stress Reduction:**

Stress is a silent saboteur of fat loss. When you're stressed, your body produces cortisol, a hormone that can promote fat storage, especially around the abdominal area. Deep, mindful breathing is an effective tool for managing stress. It triggers the relaxation response, reducing cortisol levels and creating a more favorable environment for fat loss.

**Appetite Regulation:**

Breathing mindfully can help you better regulate your appetite. When you're stressed or anxious, you're more likely to make impulsive food choices and overeat. Conscious breathing calms the mind and allows you to make more rational decisions about food, helping you avoid emotional eating and stay on track with your fat loss goals.

**Mindful Eating:**

The act of conscious breathing pairs seamlessly with mindful eating. When you're present and fully engaged with your meal, you're less likely to overindulge or make unhealthy food choices. By taking deep breaths before and during meals, you create a space for appreciation and awareness of the nourishment you're providing your body.

**Calming Cravings:**

Cravings, especially for sugary or high-calorie foods, can sabotage your fat loss efforts. Deep breathing can be a powerful tool for combating cravings. When you feel the urge to indulge, take a moment to breathe deeply. This can help you resist the temptation and make healthier choices.

**Boosting Metabolism:**

Efficient breathing can boost your metabolism. When you breathe deeply, you engage your diaphragm and stimulate the lymphatic system, which helps eliminate toxins from your body. This cleansing effect can improve your overall metabolic function, aiding in fat loss.

**Better Sleep:**

Quality sleep is crucial for fat loss and overall health. Breathing exercises, such as progressive muscle relaxation and diaphragmatic breathing, can promote relaxation and improve the quality of your sleep. Adequate rest is essential for recovery and hormonal balance, both of which support fat loss.

**Post-Workout Recovery:**

After a challenging workout, focused breathing can aid in recovery. It helps reduce post-exercise soreness and promotes relaxation, allowing your body to repair and rebuild effectively. This, in turn, can enhance your overall fitness and fat loss progress.

**Building Mind-Body Awareness:**

Fat loss is not just about physical changes but also about developing a deeper connection between your mind and body. Conscious breathing practices, such as yoga and meditation, can help you build this awareness. When you're in tune with your body's needs and signals, you're better equipped to make choices that support your fat loss goals.

**Stress-Free Consistency:**

Ultimately, the key to successful and sustainable fat loss is consistency. Breathing exercises can serve as a stress-relief tool that keeps you consistent in your fat loss journey. When you're not overwhelmed by stress, you're more likely to stick to your workout routines and healthy eating habits.

In conclusion, the importance of conscious and mindful breathing in your fat loss journey cannot be understated. It's a simple yet powerful tool that supports your metabolism, reduces stress, regulates appetite, and promotes overall well-being. By incorporating mindful breathing into your daily routine, you can enhance the effectiveness of your fat loss efforts and enjoy a healthier, more balanced approach to reaching your goals. So, take a moment to inhale deeply, exhale mindfully, and let your breath guide you towards a leaner, healthier you.

By following the link below, you will discover more about the TOOLS that can help improve your BREATHING Techniques:

bit.ly/THE10SBREATH

https://www.the10sprotocol.com/s-s-s-b

## S for STEP UP

Action is crucial in the pursuit of fat loss. It involves overcoming procrastination, eliminating excuses, and owning your health. Change starts with commitment, realistic goals, and a clear vision of your objectives, be it fat loss or healthier habits. Once committed, it's time to act. Planning workouts or meals ahead can spur momentum and a sense of achievement.

Accountability also plays a critical role; help from professionals, support groups, or accountability partners can provide the encouragement and motivation you need. Embracing fat loss often means leaving your comfort zone, trying new things and pushing harder during workouts, all of which accelerate progress towards your goals.

Consistency in making daily healthy choices, even when tough, helps cultivate lifelong habits. Simultaneously, self-care—tending to your physical, mental, and emotional well-being—is paramount. Prioritizing adequate sleep, stress management, and enjoyable pastimes can reduce stress and boost your commitment to fat loss.

Essentially, embracing fat loss requires a mindset shift, a sense of responsibility for your wellness, and positive lifestyle changes. While the fat loss journey can be challenging, by staying dedicated, positive, and proactive, you can overcome hurdles. Commitment, action, accountability, stepping outside your comfort zone, consistency, and self-care are keys to success in fat loss. Your focus, positivity, and resilience will guide you towards a healthier, happier life.

## S for STRESS

I have written a book called the 10S PROTOCOL where I emphasize 10 points in particular that are crucial for an effective fat loss. STRESS is one of the 10S.

In the pursuit of a leaner and healthier body, stress is often regarded as an abstract villain lurking in the shadows, rarely given the attention it deserves. Yet, the importance of stress in the context of fat loss cannot be overstated. Stress is not merely a mental and emotional state; it's a physiological response that can profoundly affect your body's ability to shed unwanted fat. Let's unravel the complex relationship between stress and fat loss and why managing stress is crucial for your success.

### The Stress Hormone: Cortisol

At the heart of the stress-fat loss connection is the hormone cortisol. Often referred to as the "stress hormone," cortisol is released by your adrenal glands in response to stress, whether it's physical, emotional, or psychological. While cortisol serves important functions in the body, prolonged or excessive exposure to it can lead to several fat loss roadblocks.

### Fat Storage, especially in the Abdomen:

Cortisol promotes the storage of fat, particularly in the abdominal area. This type of fat, known as visceral fat, is not only stubborn but also linked to an increased risk of various health issues, including cardiovascular disease and insulin resistance. So, when you're stressed, your body is more prone to accumulating fat, making it harder to lose those extra pounds.

### Muscle Loss:

Cortisol can lead to muscle breakdown. This is a significant concern because muscle is metabolically active tissue that helps burn calories, even at rest. When cortisol levels are chronically elevated, it can hinder your ability to maintain and build muscle, which, in turn, affects your metabolism and fat loss efforts.

### Increased Cravings for High-Calorie Foods:

Emotional or stress-induced eating is a common response to elevated cortisol levels. Stress can trigger cravings, often for sugary, high-calorie comfort foods. Giving in to these cravings can lead to overeating and a surplus of calories, making fat loss more challenging.

### Inefficient Fat Burning:

Stress can impair the body's ability to burn fat for energy. It shifts your metabolism towards using carbohydrates instead. This means that even if you're eating a calorie deficit and exercising, your body might not efficiently tap into fat stores for fuel, stalling your fat loss progress.

### Disrupted Sleep:

Chronic stress can lead to sleep disturbances, including insomnia and poor sleep quality. Inadequate sleep has a direct impact on hormones that regulate appetite and metabolism, making it more difficult to control your food intake and manage your weight.

### Emotional Eating and Binge Eating:

Stress can trigger emotional eating, a behavior where individuals turn to food as a way to cope with stress, anxiety, or other negative emotions. Binge eating, which often accompanies emotional eating, can significantly hinder fat loss progress due to the excessive calorie intake associated with it.

### Exercise and Recovery Challenges:

Stress affects your exercise routine and recovery as well. Overtraining, common among individuals experiencing high stress levels, can lead to injury and muscle fatigue. Additionally, the lack of proper recovery due to stress can impede your workout performance and overall fitness progress.

**Managing Stress for Successful Fat Loss:**

The significance of stress management in your fat loss journey cannot be emphasized enough. Here are some strategies to mitigate stress and optimize your efforts:

- **Mindfulness and Relaxation Techniques:** Engage in practices such as meditation, deep breathing, and yoga to reduce stress levels.

- **Regular Physical Activity:** Exercise is a powerful stress-reduction tool. Incorporate regular workouts into your routine to help manage stress effectively.

- **Adequate Sleep:** Prioritize quality sleep to support hormone balance and overall well-being.

- **Balanced Nutrition:** A well-balanced diet rich in nutrient-dense foods can help your body cope with stress more effectively.

- **Seeking Support:** Don't hesitate to reach out to friends, family, or a mental health professional if you're experiencing chronic stress that's affecting your fat loss journey.

In conclusion, stress is a formidable obstacle on the path to fat loss. Its impact on hormones, cravings, and metabolism can make shedding unwanted pounds an uphill battle. However, by prioritizing stress management and adopting healthy coping mechanisms, you can optimize your body's fat-burning potential and enhance your overall well-being. Recognize the importance of managing stress as an essential component of your fat loss strategy, and watch as your efforts yield more sustainable and rewarding results.

By following the link below, you will discover more about the TOOLS that can help improve your STRESS Management:

https://bit.ly/THE10SMEDITATION

https://www.the10sprotocol.com/stress

## S for STRETCHING

I have written a book called the 10S PROTOCOL where I emphasize 10 points in particular that are crucial for an effective fat loss. STRETCHING is one of the 10S.

When it comes to losing fat, most people immediately think of diet and exercise. While these factors are undeniably crucial, there's another often-overlooked component that can significantly impact your fat loss journey: stretching. The importance of stretching extends far beyond flexibility; it plays a vital role in your body's ability to burn fat efficiently. Let's delve into why stretching is a secret weapon for effective fat loss.

**Enhanced Muscle Function:**

Stretching promotes better muscle function, which is essential for fat loss. When your muscles are supple and flexible, they can contract more efficiently during exercise. This means you can engage your muscles more effectively during workouts, leading to improved calorie burn and fat loss.

**Improved Posture and Alignment:**

Poor posture and misalignment can hinder your ability to perform exercises correctly, reducing their effectiveness. Stretching helps improve posture and alignment by elongating tight muscles and releasing tension. As a result, you can engage the right muscles during workouts, maximizing your calorie expenditure and fat-burning potential.

**Injury Prevention:**

Injuries can be a major setback in your fat loss journey. Stretching plays a crucial role in injury prevention by enhancing the flexibility of muscles and joints. When your body is more limber, you're less likely to strain or injure yourself during exercise, allowing you to stay consistent with your fat loss workouts.

**Reduction of Muscle Imbalances:**

Muscle imbalances, where some muscles are stronger or tighter than others, can disrupt your body's movement patterns and lead to inefficient workouts. Stretching helps address these imbalances, ensuring that all muscles contribute to your exercise efforts. This balanced muscle engagement enhances your fat-burning potential.

**Stress Reduction:**

Stress is a known obstacle to fat loss. Chronic stress can elevate cortisol levels, promoting fat storage and hindering fat burning. Stretching, particularly practices like yoga and Pilates, can serve as a form of stress relief. It helps calm the mind, reduce cortisol levels, and create a more conducive environment for fat loss.

**Enhanced Range of Motion:**

Effective fat loss workouts often require a full range of motion. Stretching increases your range of motion, enabling you to perform exercises with proper form and greater intensity. This translates to more calories burned and more fat lost during each workout.

**Post-Workout Recovery:**

Stretching is an integral part of the post-workout cool-down process. It helps your body transition from a state of exertion to relaxation. Gentle stretching after exercise can alleviate muscle soreness and reduce the risk of stiffness, ensuring that you're ready for your next fat-burning workout.

**Mind-Body Connection:**

Stretching is not just about physical flexibility; it also promotes a mind-body connection. It encourages you to tune in to your body, become more aware of its needs, and make mindful choices regarding your exercise and nutrition. This heightened awareness can help you stay committed to your fat loss goals.

Incorporating stretching into your fat loss routine doesn't have to be time-consuming or complicated. Simple stretches before and after workouts, or even during breaks throughout the day, can yield significant benefits. Whether you choose static stretching, dynamic stretching, or a combination of both, remember that flexibility and mobility are not just about reaching your toes; they're about unlocking your body's potential for efficient fat burning.

In conclusion, stretching is a secret weapon in your fat loss arsenal. It enhances muscle function, reduces the risk of injury, improves posture, and fosters a mind-body connection that can keep you on track with your fat loss goals. So, before you embark on your next workout, take a moment to stretch and unlock your body's full potential for fat loss success.

By following the link below, you will discover more about the TOOLS that can help improve your STRETCHING Techniques:

https://www.the10sprotocol.com/stretching

## S for SUGAR & SALT

I have written a book called the 10S PROTOCOL where I emphasize 10 points in particular that are crucial for an effective fat loss. Sugar & Salt is one of the 10S.

In the complex world of fat loss, two dietary components often stand at the center of attention: sugar and salt. These two ingredients have a profound impact on our taste buds, our health, and our ability to shed unwanted pounds. Understanding the importance of sugar and salt in your fat loss journey is essential for making informed dietary choices and achieving sustainable results.

**Sugar: The Sweet Temptation**

Sugar, with its enticing sweetness, often finds its way into our diets in various forms, from table sugar to high-fructose corn syrup hidden in processed foods. While sugar itself is not inherently evil, its excessive consumption can sabotage your fat loss efforts in several ways.

**Excess Calories:**

The most direct way sugar impacts fat loss is by adding extra calories to your diet. Sugary foods and drinks are typically calorie-dense but provide little nutritional value. When you consume more calories than your body needs, the excess is stored as fat, hindering your fat loss goals.

## Blood Sugar Roller Coaster:

High-sugar foods can lead to rapid spikes and crashes in blood sugar levels. When your blood sugar drops, you're more likely to experience intense cravings and hunger, making it challenging to control your calorie intake and maintain a healthy eating plan.

## Insulin Resistance:

Consistently high sugar intake can lead to insulin resistance, a condition where your cells become less responsive to insulin, a hormone that regulates blood sugar. Insulin resistance is associated with weight gain, particularly around the abdomen, making fat loss more difficult.

## Promoting Fat Storage:

Excess sugar can promote the storage of fat, especially in the liver. When the liver is overwhelmed with sugar, it converts it into fat for storage. This can contribute to fatty liver disease and make it harder to burn existing body fat.

## Cravings for More Sugar:

Consuming sugar triggers the release of dopamine, a feel-good neurotransmitter. This can create a cycle of sugar cravings, as your brain associates sugar with pleasure. These cravings can lead to overconsumption and hinder your fat loss progress.

## SALT: THE SNEAKY CULPRIT

Salt, or sodium, is an essential mineral that our bodies need to function properly. However, excessive salt intake can have detrimental effects on fat loss and overall health.

## Water Retention:

High salt intake can cause your body to retain water. This can lead to temporary weight gain, making it challenging to track your fat loss progress and causing frustration.

### Increased Appetite:

Salty foods can stimulate your appetite. When you consume high-salt meals, you may find yourself eating more calories than you intended, which can impede your fat loss efforts.

### Health Risks:

A diet high in salt is associated with an increased risk of hypertension (high blood pressure) and cardiovascular disease. These health issues can make exercise and fat loss more challenging.

### Cravings for Salty Foods:

Just as sugar triggers cravings, salt can also stimulate a desire for more salty foods. This can lead to a cycle of overconsumption, making it difficult to stick to a balanced diet.

### Finding Balance:

The key to navigating the sweet and salty seas in your fat loss journey lies in finding balance. It's not necessary to eliminate sugar and salt completely from your diet, but rather to consume them in moderation and make healthier choices.

### Sugar :

- Choose natural sugars from fruits and vegetables over added sugars.
- Read food labels and limit consumption of sugary processed foods and sugary beverages.
- Be mindful of portion sizes when enjoying sweet treats.

### Salt :

- Opt for whole, unprocessed foods that are naturally lower in sodium.
- Use herbs and spices to flavor your meals instead of relying on excessive salt.

- Limit your intake of highly processed, salty foods like chips, fast food, and canned soups.

In conclusion, sugar and salt play significant roles in your fat loss journey, and understanding their impact is essential for success. While they can pose challenges, moderation and mindful choices can help you harness the benefits of these ingredients while minimizing their negative effects. By finding a balanced approach to sugar and salt in your diet, you can navigate the scas of fat loss with confidence, making steady progress toward your goals while preserving your long-term health.

## S for SUPPLEMENT

I have written a book called the 10S PROTOCOL where I emphasize 10 points in particular that are crucial for an effective fat loss. Supplement is one of the 10S.

In the ever-evolving world of health and fitness, supplements have become a topic of great interest and discussion, particularly when it comes to losing fat. Many individuals seek a magic pill or powder that promises quick and effortless fat loss. However, it's crucial to approach the topic of supplements with a discerning eye and a healthy dose of skepticism. Let's explore the role of supplements in your fat loss journey and discern what's truly important.

**Dietary Supplements vs. Magic Bullets:**

Supplements are intended to complement, not replace, a balanced and nutritious diet. It's important to understand that there is no magic pill that can miraculously melt away fat without the need for a healthy diet and regular physical activity. While some supplements may offer modest support, they are not a substitute for lifestyle changes.

**The Supplement Hype:**

The supplement industry is rife with marketing hype and sensational claims. Beware of products that promise rapid and unrealistic fat loss results. Such claims often lack scientific evidence and can lead to disappointment and frustration.

**The Importance of a Solid Foundation:**

Before considering supplements, ensure that you have established a solid foundation for fat loss through proper nutrition and exercise. Supplements should be viewed as the icing on the cake, not the cake itself. They can provide a slight edge when your fundamentals are in place.

**Types of Supplements:**

Let's take a closer look at some common types of supplements often associated with fat loss:

- **1. Protein Supplements:** Protein is essential for muscle preservation and metabolism. Protein supplements like whey protein can be beneficial if you struggle to meet your protein needs through whole foods, but they are not a magic solution for fat loss.

- **2. Fat Burners:** Fat burner supplements often contain caffeine and other ingredients that claim to increase metabolism and fat oxidation. While some may provide a temporary boost in energy, their long-term effectiveness is questionable, and they can have side effects.

- **3. Vitamins and Minerals:** Certain vitamins and minerals, such as vitamin D, calcium, and magnesium, play roles in metabolic processes. However, deficiencies should be addressed through a balanced diet rather than supplements.

**The Scientific Perspective:**

The scientific evidence regarding the effectiveness of most fat loss supplements is often inconclusive or limited. While some studies suggest potential benefits, the results are typically modest and vary among individuals. It's crucial to consult with a healthcare professional or registered dietitian before adding any supplements to your regimen.

**Safety and Side Effects:**

Supplements are not without risks. Some can interact with medications or have adverse effects. Additionally, the quality and purity of supplements vary widely, making it essential to choose reputable brands and products.

**A Holistic Approach:**

Rather than focusing solely on supplements, consider adopting a holistic approach to fat loss that includes the following elements:

- **1. Balanced Diet:** Prioritize a diet rich in whole foods, including lean proteins, fruits, vegetables, whole grains, and healthy fats.
- **2. Regular Exercise:** Combine cardiovascular workouts with resistance training to maximize fat loss and preserve lean muscle mass.
- **3. Adequate Sleep:** Quality sleep is crucial for hormone regulation and fat loss. Aim for 7-9 hours of restful sleep each night.
- **4. Stress Management:** Chronic stress can hinder fat loss efforts. Practice stress-reduction techniques like meditation, yoga, or deep breathing.
- **5. Hydration:** Staying well-hydrated supports metabolism and overall health.

**Conclusion:**

While supplements can be a part of your fat loss strategy, they should be approached with caution and used in conjunction with a well-rounded and evidence-based approach to nutrition and fitness. Remember that there is no substitute for the fundamentals of a balanced diet and regular exercise when it comes to losing fat. Seek guidance from healthcare professionals or registered dietitians to make informed decisions about supplements that may complement your fat loss journey without compromising your health or expectations.

By following the link below, you will discover more about the TOOLS that can help improve your HEALTH :

https://www.the10sprotocol.com/supplements

# T

## T for TELEVISION

While television offers entertainment, it can inadvertently hinder fat loss due to encouraging sedentary behavior, poor eating habits, and sleep disturbances. Prolonged TV viewing slows metabolism and fosters mindless consumption of unhealthy snacks, contributing to weight gain. It can also compromise sleep quality and length, with insufficient sleep linked to obesity and elevated calorie intake. The TV's blue light can disrupt natural sleep cycles, further affecting sleep.

TV content often promotes unhealthy lifestyle choices, like junk food consumption, sedentary habits, smoking, and substance use, complicating fat loss. The impact on children is particularly concerning, with those watching over two hours of TV daily showing higher tendencies toward obesity, poor dietary habits, and decreased physical activity.

Although TV isn't the sole contributor to weight gain, reducing its consumption and adopting healthier habits can mitigate its negative effects. To counter TV's impact on fat loss, limit your screen time, with the American Heart Association recommending no more than two hours daily for adults. Replace TV time with physical activities, opt for healthier snacks or avoid eating while watching TV, and ensure ample sleep by avoiding electronics before bedtime.

In conclusion, while TV watching is enjoyable, it can impede fat loss by promoting a sedentary lifestyle, poor eating, and sleep interference. To minimize these effects, regulate screen time, choose healthier snacks, get sufficient sleep, and partake in physical activity.

## T for TEMPLE

"YOUR BODY IS A GIFT FROM GOD, IT SHOULD BE PROTECTED LIKE FORT KNOX"

Your body deserves proper care for overall well-being, and a significant aspect of this is a healthy diet. More than a weight-loss strategy, a nutritious diet boosts overall health and vitality. A balanced intake of fruits, vegetables, whole grains, lean proteins, and healthy fats can reduce the risk of chronic diseases like heart disease and diabetes, and also enhance energy levels and mood.

Body respect includes being mindful of food choices. Diets rich in processed foods and unhealthy fats, which are often calorie-dense but nutrient-poor, can harm health. Conversely, nourishing your body with wholesome foods rich in vitamins, minerals, and antioxidants boosts immunity, supports organ function, and promotes health.

Mindful eating is also integral, which includes paying attention to portion sizes and responding to your body's hunger and satiety cues. Adequate hydration is essential for digestion, nutrient transport, and detoxification.

Regular physical activity is another key component in treating your body like a temple. Regular exercise improves both physical and mental health, enhances mood, reduces stress, and encourages good sleep.

In essence, treating your body as a temple means nourishing it with nutritious foods, practicing mindful eating and hydration, staying active, and caring for mental health. By honoring your body and providing it with the care it deserves, you can attain optimal health and reap its myriad benefits.

## T for TESTOSTERONE

Testosterone, a hormone crucial for muscle growth, bone density, and cognitive function, also plays a significant role in fat loss and muscle gain. This hormone is predominant in men but also present in smaller amounts in women.

One of the main advantages of testosterone is its ability to boost muscle mass by enhancing protein synthesis. It also maintains bone density, reducing fracture risk, especially in older age. In addition, testosterone aids cognitive function, including memory, concentration, and spatial abilities.

In terms of fat loss, testosterone increases metabolism, thus promoting fat loss and preventing weight gain. Low testosterone levels can result in issues like depression, fatigue, and decreased libido.

Diet can help increase testosterone levels. A diet high in protein and healthy fats, the building blocks for testosterone, is beneficial. Foods like eggs, meat, and dairy products provide cholesterol, which is used to synthesize testosterone. Certain vitamins and minerals like vitamin D, zinc, and magnesium found in greens, nuts, and seeds, are also crucial for testosterone production.

Keeping a healthy body weight is vital since excess fat can decrease testosterone levels. Besides diet, factors like exercise, stress management, and sleep also affect testosterone levels. A holistic approach to health can help maintain optimal testosterone levels.

In conclusion, diet and overall health significantly impact testosterone levels. A balanced diet rich in proteins, healthy fats, and essential nutrients can boost testosterone levels, providing benefits like muscle growth, fat loss, and improved cognitive function. A comprehensive health approach is crucial for maintaining healthy testosterone levels.

## WAYS TO INCREASE TESTOSTERONE LEVELS NATURALLY

There are several ways to increase testosterone levels naturally. Here are some of the most effective methods:

1. Exercise regularly: Engaging in regular exercise, especially strength training, has been shown to increase testosterone levels.

2. Maintain a healthy weight: Excess body fat can decrease testosterone levels, so maintaining a healthy weight through a balanced diet and regular exercise is important.

3. Get enough sleep: Sleep is crucial for hormone regulation, and studies have shown that getting enough sleep can help to increase testosterone levels.

4. Reduce stress: Chronic stress can lead to decreased testosterone levels, so managing stress through relaxation techniques like meditation, yoga, or deep breathing can be helpful.

5. Eat a healthy diet: Consuming a diet that is high in protein, healthy fats, and whole foods can help to support testosterone production. Foods rich in zinc, vitamin D, and magnesium are particularly important.

6. Take supplements: Almost all vitamins and minerals impact the level of testosterone in one way or another. Adding supplements such as zinc, vitamin D, and DHEA, have been shown to help increase testosterone levels in some people. However, it's important to speak with a healthcare provider before taking any supplements.

7. Limit alcohol consumption: Alcohol consumption can interfere with testosterone production, so limiting or avoiding alcohol may be helpful.

8. Avoid smoking: Smoking has been shown to decrease testosterone levels, so quitting smoking can be beneficial for overall health and hormone balance.

9. Improve your posture. Studies have shown that improving your posture helped produce more testosterone just because having a better posture helped decrease the level of cortisol which is a testosterone blocker.

10. Reduce your exposure to man-made chemicals.

11. Get enough good fat food.

12. Ginger root. It has shown that consuming ginger daily for 90 days was able to increase testosterone level by 17%. You should consume around 1 to 3 grams a day of it.

13. Have a visit to your physician. Indeed, sometimes the low level of testosterone has a physical origin, like Varicoceles which is an obstruction of the canal (vein) coming from your testicle, preventing the testosterone from being distributed. Of course, a healthy lifestyle can improve and cure this problem but not all the time. This problem is common, it touches 15% of the population. Which is a lot. So don't be ashamed to go and get it checked out.

Last but not least is Tongkat Ali.

Tongkat Ali, also known as Eurycoma longifolia or Malaysian ginseng, is a flowering plant native to Southeast Asia. It has been used for centuries in traditional medicine to treat a variety of conditions, including infertility, erectile dysfunction, and low energy levels.

The root of the Tongkat Ali plant is typically used for medicinal purposes, and it is believed to contain several active compounds that may have beneficial effects on the body. One of these compounds is called eurycomanone, which has been shown to have antioxidant and anti-inflammatory properties.

Tongkat Ali is also proven to affect testosterone levels in the body. Some research has proven that it helps to increase testosterone production, which can lead to improvements in libido, muscle mass, and energy levels.

A Study has shown an increase of +37% in 4 weeks and a decrease of cortisol level of 16% by taking 200 mg of that herb. To be effective, you should take 200 to 300 mg (because of your overweight) of the 100:1 extract concentration.

By following this link, you will find the best and cleanest Tongkat Ali in the market:

https://www.the10sprotocol.com/supplements

Another natural supplement that can be very helpful is Forskolin.

Forskolin is a natural compound found in the roots of the Indian coleus plant (Coleus Forskohlii). It has been used in traditional Ayurvedic medicine for centuries to treat a variety of health conditions, including high blood pressure, chest pain, and respiratory disorders.

Forskolin is believed to work by increasing levels of a molecule called cyclic adenosine monophosphate (cAMP) in the body. This molecule is involved in many biological processes, including the regulation of glucose and lipid metabolism, the relaxation of smooth muscle tissue, and the stimulation of hormone production.

One of the most well-known benefits of forskolin is its potential ability to promote fat loss. Some studies have suggested that forskolin may help to increase metabolism and promote fat breakdown, leading to reductions in body weight and body fat percentage.

Another study has shown that people who took 250 mg of 10% Forskolin twice a day have seen their level increase by 33%.

By following this link, you will find the best and cleanest Forskolin in the market:

https://www.the10sprotocol.com/supplements

It's important to note that while these natural methods can help increase testosterone levels, they may not be effective for everyone. If you are experiencing symptoms of low testosterone, such as decreased libido, fatigue, or muscle weakness, it's important to speak with a healthcare provider to determine the underlying cause and develop an appropriate treatment plan.

## T for THERAPY

Starting a diet can be tough, but therapy can provide valuable support. Therapy helps identify and tackle emotional and psychological factors that drive unhealthy eating. For instance, if you turn to food to relieve stress, therapy can assist in developing healthier coping strategies.

Therapy provides ongoing support and accountability, crucial for maintaining diet and exercise plans. Working with a therapist, you can set clear goals and form strategies to achieve them. Regular sessions can celebrate successes and troubleshoot issues that come up.

Body image issues often fuel unhealthy eating. Therapy can help challenge these negative perceptions and cultivate a positive relationship with your body, promoting a healthier approach to fat loss. It's important to remember that this journey isn't just about losing weight but also about self-acceptance and self-love.

Group therapy and support groups can offer a sense of community and shared experiences. However, therapy isn't a one-size-fits-all solution. Different approaches, like cognitive-behavioral or mindfulness-based therapy, might suit different individuals.

Ultimately, successful dieting hinges on finding the right support and resources. Therapy can help manage emotional or psychological issues contributing to unhealthy eating habits. Whether dealing with stress eating, body image issues, or other challenges, therapy can equip you with the skills needed for lasting success.

## T for THINK

Dieting can be complex and requires careful planning. Success is dependent on making informed decisions about food selection and timing, based on realistic expectations and personal goals. To begin, understanding your body's requirements is key. Consider your daily calorie, macronutrient and micronutrient needs, along with any health conditions that might influence your diet. Select nutrient-dense foods such as fruits, vegetables, lean proteins, and whole grains over processed, sugary options.

Portion control is critical. Even healthy foods can lead to weight gain if consumed excessively. Pay attention to serving sizes, and listen to your body's hunger and fullness signals.

Your lifestyle factors into your diet too. If you're busy, meal prep can ensure you have nutritious choices on hand. If socializing often involves food, consider how your diet can accommodate these situations.

Mental and emotional health play a crucial role in dieting, which can sometimes cause stress, deprivation or guilt. To counter this, create a support network of friends, family, or professionals like dietitians. Embrace self-care and positivity, particularly during challenges.

In essence, successful dieting combines informed food choices, portion control, lifestyle considerations, and emotional health. With a strong support system and a forgiving approach to setbacks, you can attain your health goals and maintain a positive relationship with food and your body.

## T for TIME

**"WHOEVER MASTERS HIS/HER TIME MASTERS HIS/HER LIFE."**

THE IMPORTANCE OF TIME HORIZON

In the world of dieting, time is often overlooked. People tend to focus on food and exercise, forgetting that fat loss requires time, patience, and realistic expectations. Rushing to see results can lead to harmful practices like crash diets.

A routine is essential in managing time effectively. Consistency in meal planning, exercise schedules, and sleep patterns helps foster long-term healthy habits, preventing unhealthy choices and missed workouts.

Over time, healthy habits such as meal prepping, regular exercise, and sufficient sleep become ingrained, leading to sustainable lifestyle changes. Time also allows for personal experimentation - through trial and error, you can discover what works best for your body.

Moreover, long-term benefits of time in dieting shouldn't be ignored. Quick-fix diets might deliver fast results, but they're often not sustainable. By focusing on long-term goals and gradual changes, you can achieve better, lasting results. The progress might be slow, but it's more sustainable.

Finally, despite life's demands, time should be dedicated to health, as it can boost energy, productivity, and overall well-being.

In conclusion, time is a key player in dieting. It allows for sustainable habits, personal discoveries, and patience. Prioritizing time for health can lead to long-term success. Remember, consistency, patience, and time commitment to health are worth it in the end.

## MANAGING TIME ON A DAILY BASIS

Balancing a healthy diet with work, family, and other commitments can be daunting, but effective time management is pivotal for success. Here's why :

1. **Creating a schedule**: Pre-planning meals prevents unhealthy, last-minute choices. With a meal schedule, you're prepared with necessary ingredients, evading the lure of fast food.

2. **Prioritizing activities**: Time management helps prioritize vital activities like exercise, cooking, and meal planning, ensuring sufficient time allocation to maintain a healthy diet.

3. **Sticking to a routine**: A routine, facilitated by good time management, can include specified slots for exercise, meal planning, grocery shopping, and cooking. Such structure aids in sustaining healthy choices.

4. **Reducing stress**: Knowing you've allotted time for necessary tasks reduces diet-related stress. Lower stress levels increase adherence to your diet plan and deter unhealthy choices.

5. **Increasing productivity**: Effective time management boosts productivity by allowing more to be accomplished in less time, freeing up space for exercise, meal planning, and other health-focused activities.

6. **Achieving goals**: Time management aids in achieving diet goals. Dedicating time for health-promoting activities ensures you adhere to your diet plan, thus meeting your

targets. Enhanced productivity also allows more achievement in less time.

7. **Building healthy habits**: A routine that incorporates exercise, meal planning, and other healthy activities fosters long-lasting habits, promoting sustained healthy living.

Time management is crucial for successful dieting, aiding in establishing routines, reducing stress, improving productivity, and forming healthy habits. It requires a committed mindset to achieve dieting goals. But remember, your time is valuable. Prioritizing others over your health can jeopardize your diet, exercise regime, and overall goal. It's essential not to neglect your health while helping others. Sometimes saying no is vital. Choosing yourself first is a simple but important step in managing time effectively and successfully pursuing your health goals.

## T for TOXICITY

IN YOUR LIFE

Initiating a diet comes with its challenges, often amplified by toxic elements in life, such as negative relationships, unsupportive environments, harmful habits, and stress eating.

Toxic relationships can lead to emotional distress and unhealthy eating, so addressing them is crucial for mental well-being and diet success. Environments riddled with stress can trigger poor eating habits, making a supportive and decluttered surrounding essential.

Harmful habits like excessive smoking or drinking impair both physical and mental health, undermining dieting efforts. Developing healthy mechanisms for coping with stress and emotions, such as mindfulness or regular exercise, is pivotal in reducing harmful eating behaviors.

Having a circle of positive influences, perhaps through supportive friends, family, diet groups, or a dietitian, provides additional motivation and guidance.

In essence, tackling life's toxicity, embracing positivity, adopting healthy coping mechanisms, and seeking support when needed can overcome barriers to a healthy diet, leading to improved overall health and well-being.

## IN YOUR BODY

Starting a diet is a significant step, and internal factors, particularly bodily toxicity, play a crucial role in your success. Bodily toxicity can emerge from an unhealthy diet, exposure to environmental toxins, and physical inactivity, each posing significant health concerns that can derail dieting efforts.

A diet high in processed foods, sugars, and bad fats triggers inflammation and digestive issues while increasing unhealthy food cravings. Environmental toxins, found in air, water, and everyday items, can cause fatigue, headaches, and a weakened immune system.

Additionally, a sedentary lifestyle hinders your body's toxin-elimination process, leading to health issues like fatigue, weight gain, and weakened immunity.

Therefore, starting a diet requires adopting changes that promote detoxification and overall health. Incorporate nutrient-rich foods in your diet, reduce environmental toxin exposure, and engage in regular physical activities to support body detoxification.

Further, hydration, sufficient sleep, and stress management support your body's natural detoxification process and overall well-being.

To sum up, tackling bodily toxicity – caused by an unhealthy diet, environmental toxins, and physical inactivity – through lifestyle changes that promote detoxification and health, is essential for successful dieting and achieving optimal health and wellness.

## T for TOXIN

Starting a diet calls for a comprehensive approach to health, which must include reducing toxins. Our bodies encounter harmful substances via environmental pollution, processed food, and stress, negatively impacting our cells and organs, leading to weight gain, inflammation, and hormonal imbalances. When dieting, we must first lessen this toxic burden.

Identify toxin sources around you such as polluted air, cleaning product chemicals, and non-organic foods. Actively choose to lower your exposure by picking natural cleaning products and organic foods.

It's also crucial to strengthen your body's detox abilities. Aid your liver and kidneys, the toxin-eliminating organs, by eating nutrient- and antioxidant-rich foods like leafy greens, berries, and cruciferous vegetables.

Remember, chronic stress can spike cortisol levels, causing inflammation and other health issues. Thus, incorporate relaxation methods like meditation, deep breathing, or yoga daily. Seek expert advice for more stress management strategies if needed.

Getting enough sleep is vital as it enables your body to repair and detoxify. Aim for 7-8 hours nightly and keep a regular sleep schedule.

In short, managing toxins is key when starting a diet. By lowering toxin exposure, enhancing body detoxification, controlling stress, and sleeping adequately, you'll better your health and wellness. Give your body the care it deserves.

## T for TRANSCENDENCE

Fat loss is more than just a physical pursuit; it's also a mental and emotional journey, encapsulated in the concept of transcendence. Transcendence involves surpassing current habits, thoughts, and emotions, and it's essential for lasting fat loss and improved well-being.

Transcendence in fat loss can manifest in several ways. Mindfulness is one approach, where fully immersing in the present moment enhances awareness of hunger and fullness signals, encouraging healthier eating habits.

Transcendence also involves examining and confronting limiting beliefs and negative self-talk that keep us stuck in unhealthy patterns. Recognizing and challenging these perspectives allows for the development of a more positive, empowering mindset.

Finding deeper meaning and purpose in your fat loss journey is another aspect of transcendence. Whether it's a desire for longevity or wanting to be a positive role model, these values can inspire commitment to your fat loss goals.

The act of surrendering, or relinquishing the need to control every detail of the journey, is also a part of transcendence. Accepting the inevitable fluctuations of fat loss can reduce stress and increase the chances of long-term success.

Achieving transcendence in fat loss requires patience, resilience, and the courage to confront obstructive beliefs and habits. The benefits are considerable, encompassing improved physical health, heightened self-awareness, and a richer sense of purpose and meaning.

A supportive community can facilitate the cultivation of transcendence in fat loss. Whether it's a support group, therapy, or like-minded friends and family, encouragement from others can significantly boost motivation.

In conclusion, embracing transcendence can significantly enhance long-term fat loss and overall well-being. By practicing mindfulness, challenging limiting beliefs, aligning with deeper values, and accepting the journey's natural flow, you can achieve transformative changes that go beyond fat loss. You can create a more fulfilling, purposeful life. If you're ready to elevate your fat loss journey, consider the power of transcendence.

## T for TRICK & TIPS

Embarking on a diet can be daunting, but certain strategies can simplify the process and enhance its effectiveness. Here are ten key tips for successful dieting :

1. Develop a plan: Define your goals, the foods you'll eat, and your progress-tracking methods before starting. A clear plan boosts motivation and focus, making adherence easier.

2. Practice mindful eating: Pay attention to your food, its taste, and how it makes you feel. Mindfulness during meals improves awareness of hunger and fullness cues, enabling healthier choices.

3. Make healthy swaps: Replace unhealthy foods with healthier alternatives. This could mean choosing whole-grain bread over white, or drinking water or herbal tea instead of sugary drinks.

4. Stay hydrated: Drink at least 8-10 glasses of water daily. Hydration helps maintain satiety, supporting your dieting efforts. Make it enjoyable by adding fruit slices or herbs.

5. Use smaller plates: smaller plates can assist in portion control. People tend to eat more when larger portions are offered, so smaller plates can mitigate this issue.

6. Keep healthy snacks on hand: Stave off the temptation of unhealthy foods by keeping healthy snacks like fresh fruit, raw vegetables, nuts, and seeds within reach.

7. Get adequate sleep: Aim for 7-8 hours of sleep each night. Insufficient sleep can trigger increased hunger and cravings, hindering dieting efforts.

8. Find an accountability partner: Someone who holds you accountable, like a friend, family member, or a dietitian, can provide helpful support during your dieting journey.

9. Practice self-compassion: Dieting can be tough, so focus on progress rather than perfection. Be kind to yourself and remember that occasional slip-ups are a normal part of the journey.

10. Be patient: Dieting is a process that takes time. Trust this process, understanding that small changes can eventually lead to significant health improvements.

In conclusion, starting a diet can be challenging, but using strategies like mindful eating, healthy swaps, and finding accountability can help you achieve your goals. Patience, self-compassion, and trust in the process are vital. With these tips, you'll be well-equipped to succeed in your dieting journey and achieve a healthier version of yourself.

## T for TRIGGERS

Starting a diet involves more than just changing what you eat; it also means understanding and addressing the triggers that can lead you astray. Triggers could be environmental, social, or emotional, and they can provoke unhealthy eating habits, potentially derailing your progress.

Environmental triggers come from your physical surroundings, such as the availability of unhealthy foods or lack of healthier alternatives. Tackling these can involve carrying healthy snacks with you or steering clear of specific environments.

Social triggers can be due to peer pressure or social events with unhealthy food options. Balancing enjoyment with dietary goals may require expressing your dietary intentions to your social circle to help mitigate these triggers.

Emotional triggers relate to how feelings influence eating habits, with deep-rooted emotional issues often playing a role. This might involve using food as a coping mechanism for stress or anxiety, and addressing them can benefit from professional help like therapy or counseling.

Along with addressing triggers, it's important to cultivate healthy stress-coping mechanisms, such as exercise or meditation. Additionally, a supportive network of family, friends, or support groups can provide invaluable encouragement.

Managing diet triggers is an ongoing process, needing self-awareness, commitment, and patience. Remember, setbacks are part of the journey, and each new day offers another opportunity to make healthier choices.

In conclusion, recognizing and managing diet triggers is vital for sustaining a healthy diet and achieving long-term success. This involves fostering healthy coping mechanisms, establishing a robust support system, and potentially seeking professional assistance. With self-awareness, dedication, and resilience, you can overcome diet hurdles and achieve your long-term health goals.

## T for TRUSTING THE PROCESS

Starting a diet typically brings a sense of excitement for quick results. However, real change takes time, making it essential to 'trust the process.' This phrase signifies understanding that results may not appear instantly, but consistent efforts will eventually yield progress. It calls for faith in oneself, the selected plan, patience, and an ability to learn from setbacks.

Many falter on diets due to lack of trust in the process. When rapid results don't materialize, they might feel disheartened and quit before their bodies adjust to the new routine. During the early detox stage, understanding that temporary discomfort like headaches or irritability are part of the adjustment process is crucial.

Trusting the process also involves setting realistic goals. Ambitious goals can lead to early discouragement if progress seems slow. It's more beneficial to establish manageable targets to maintain motivation.

Having a support network of friends, family, or a support group is invaluable. They provide motivation and help you stay on course when times get tough.

Remember, each person's journey is different. Trusting the process means remaining open to trying different strategies until you find what suits you best. Celebrating even small progress, like sticking to your meal plan for a week, boosts motivation and solidifies trust in the process.

In conclusion, trusting the dieting process requires faith, realistic goal-setting, a supportive network, and a willingness to experiment. With trust, patience, and perseverance, you can achieve your health and fitness goals, leading to a healthier, more fulfilled life.

# U

## U for UNFAIR

The world of diet and fitness showcases a stark reality: body types aren't created equal. Some individuals, gifted with fast metabolisms, find weight maintenance easier than others who struggle despite sincere efforts due to slower metabolic rates. This disparity often fuels frustration and can make people give up their health aspirations. It's crucial to recognize that these differences are largely uncontrollable, rendering comparisons unproductive and unfair.

The media often intensifies this issue by promoting unrealistic beauty norms, triggering body image insecurities and unhealthy diet habits. Societal pressure to conform to specific body types can induce harmful practices like crash dieting, overexercising, and disordered eating.

Instead, we need to emphasize personal health and well-being, acknowledging and accepting our individualities. Accepting our unique body types and metabolic capacities allows us to develop sustainable diet and fitness plans tailored to our needs. The focus should be overall wellness rather than merely targeting fat loss.

Moreover, we must challenge the social and cultural factors perpetuating body inequality. By questioning unrealistic beauty standards and celebrating diversity, we can stimulate change. Universal access to healthy food and resources, independent of socioeconomic status, is essential.

In essence, inherent body type inequality is a disappointing reality in dieting and fitness. However, it's crucial to embrace our unique bodies and metabolic rates, focusing on overall health rather than fitting a specific body mold. We should challenge unattainable beauty norms, promote diversity, and ensure everyone has access to healthy living resources. With health and wellness as the priority, we can foster a more equal society.

# V

## V for VEGETABLES

Vegetables are a must-have for a nutritious diet, overflowing with nutrients, vitamins, and minerals essential for peak health. With their low-calorie, high-fiber properties, they satisfy hunger without leading to overeating, supporting weight control. They house antioxidants that protect cells from free radicals' harmful effects, safeguarding vital molecules like DNA. Key nutrients from veggies such as vitamins C, A, K, and minerals like potassium, magnesium, iron, fortify the immune system, foster bone health, and ensure the body's smooth functioning.

Notably, vegetables are fiber powerhouses, maintaining digestive well-being and warding off issues like constipation. A diverse vegetable intake can help stave off chronic conditions like heart disease, stroke, and cancer. Studies show veggie-rich diets lower blood pressure, reduce inflammation, and enhance cardiovascular health. Vegetables' adaptability is an added bonus. They can be enjoyed raw, cooked, or even grilled and used in a variety of dishes.

In addition to being cost-effective and widely available, vegetables are environmentally friendly, demanding fewer resources for growth and thus curbing greenhouse gas emissions. To sum up, incorporating a range of vegetables in daily meals can manage weight, fend off chronic diseases, improve digestion, and provide vital nutrients, steering us towards a more vibrant, healthier lifestyle.

## V for VICTORY

Winning at fat loss is a personalized journey, where the goalposts range from target weights or sizes to improved self-esteem. Celebrating these victories can fuel motivation and boost a sense of accomplishment. A successful fat loss journey hinges on setting attainable, progressive goals, such as enhancing your daily intake of fruits and vegetables, or gradually increasing your step count. Achieving these smaller targets motivates you to stay focused on the ultimate goal.

During your journey, it's important to appreciate your progress and celebrate your wins. By rewarding yourself, whether through a new workout outfit or a healthy meal with friends, you keep your motivation up and your gaze fixed on the final objective.

Getting the right support and guidance is also crucial. A personal trainer, nutritionist, support group, or an accountability partner can offer much-needed motivation, help keep you accountable, and create a supportive space for sharing your journey.

Fat loss isn't just a physical change—it also involves mental and emotional shifts. Cultivating a healthier relationship with food and exercise, heeding your body's cues, finding physical activities you enjoy, and fostering a positive body image and self-esteem contribute to sustainable fat loss.

The journey to fat loss victory requires dedication, resilience, and self-compassion. It's okay to experience setbacks and ask for help. By setting feasible goals, applauding achievements, seeking support, and focusing on both the physical and mental facets of fat loss, you can achieve your desired outcome and evolve into your best self. This journey to success is paved with commitment, positivity, and consistent celebration of victories.

## V for VIRTUOUS CIRCLE

A virtuous circle represents a beneficial cycle where favorable actions yield more positive outcomes. In diet and nutrition, it's a chain reaction where healthy eating and consistent exercise spur advantageous body changes, encouraging healthier choices and more physical activity. The perks are wide-ranging, impacting both physical and mental health. Consuming nutritious foods and maintaining regular exercise can induce positive physical changes such as fat loss, improved cardiovascular health, and increased muscle tone, leading to lower risk of chronic diseases, boosted energy levels, and an enhanced quality of life.

Mental health also benefits from this virtuous circle. Exercise releases mood-lifting endorphins, while a wholesome diet provides vital nutrients for brain function, contributing to improved mental health. This positive cycle can bolster self-esteem and confidence. Making healthier lifestyle changes can increase your faith in your ability to make good decisions, creating a feedback loop that lifts self-confidence.

A virtuous circle can even extend its benefits socially. Healthy habits can enhance energy levels and engagement, fostering social interactions and connections, and may inspire others, causing a positive ripple in your social circle.

Constructing a virtuous circle demands dedication but yields rich rewards. Despite potential setbacks, focusing on positive changes can boost physical and mental health, self-esteem, and create a positive societal impact.

## V for VISUALIZATION

Visualization, or mental imagery, is a potent tool for accomplishing fat loss and healthier lifestyle objectives. It leverages mental images of desired outcomes to boost motivation, willpower, and dieting success.

Visualization is instrumental in surmounting mental hurdles that obstruct healthy choices. By replacing negative self-talk and limiting beliefs with images of a fit, healthy, and confident self, it encourages a positive self-image, elevates motivation, self-esteem, and instills a sense of control over health.

Visualization can help establish and achieve specific dietary goals. For instance, envisioning oneself running a 5K, fitting into favorite jeans, or feeling energetic and confident in social scenarios can sustain commitment and motivation towards fat loss goals.

Moreover, visualization can alleviate stress and anxiety associated with dieting, promoting relaxation and well-being during emotionally challenging times. Physically, it can improve athletic performance, boost muscle strength, and speed up healing post-injuries.

Visualization thrives on regular practice, which could involve daily dedicated time or incorporating it into routine activities like creating a vision board or using positive affirmations.

In conclusion, visualization is a powerful asset for anyone striving to improve their diet and achieve fat loss goals. By focusing on positive outcomes and mental images of success, it boosts motivation, reduces stress, and fosters a positive mindset that encourages healthy choices and behaviors.

## V for VITAMINS

A healthy diet goes beyond calorie-counting, also focusing on essential vitamins and minerals vital for overall health. Vitamins, required in small quantities, are crucial for various bodily functions, and deficiencies can adversely impact health.

Water-soluble vitamins, such as C and B vitamins, aren't stored in the body and need daily replenishment. These vitamins are essential for energy metabolism, immune and nerve function. Deficiencies, though rare, can occur due to restricted food intake or certain medical conditions.

Fat-soluble vitamins, namely A, D, E, and K, are stored in the body's fat tissues. They're critical for vision, immune function, and bone health. However, overconsumption can be harmful.

Vitamins enhance your immune system. Vitamins A, C, and E are antioxidants that protect cells from damage, while vitamin D aids immune function and bone health. Deficiencies can weaken the immune system, elevating illness risk.

Vitamins also promote healthy skin, hair, and nails. Vitamins A, C, E contribute to skin health, while B vitamins, especially biotin, are vital for healthy hair and nails.

Vitamins also support healthy bones. Vitamin D facilitates calcium absorption and bone growth, with calcium and vitamin K maintaining bone health.

Getting sufficient vitamins is critical, but moderation and adherence to recommended intake guidelines are important. The optimal source of vitamins is a varied diet of whole foods. Supplements can complement but should not replace a healthy diet.

In conclusion, vitamins play a crucial role in bodily functions, overall health, and wellness, promoting a robust immune system, healthy skin, hair, nails, and preventing bone loss.

By following this link, you will find the one of the most effective and cleanest Vitamins in the market:

https://www.the10sprotocol.com/supplements

## V for VOICE

On a diet, it's common to struggle with an internal negative voice that fuels self-doubt and jeopardizes progress towards fat loss and healthier eating. It's crucial to mute this inner critic to stay motivated and goal-oriented.

Firstly, identify when this negative voice arises, paying heed to thoughts during difficult moments. Replacing these negative ideas with positive self-talk is crucial.

Positive affirmations are powerful for quelling the inner critic. Statements like "I can achieve my goals," "I deserve to feel my best," and "I am worthy of a healthy life" aid in reshaping subconscious beliefs and enhancing motivation.

Also, shift focus from perfection to progress. Concentrate on small victories rather than an unrealistic ideal of perfection. This positive reinforcement boosts motivation and self-confidence, quieting the inner critic.

Practicing self-compassion is equally essential. Treating oneself with kindness during setbacks helps mute the inner critic and encourages self-acceptance.

Lastly, surround yourself with positivity. Engage with supportive communities, uplifting literature, podcasts, or positive social media to foster a healthy mindset and keep the inner critic at bay.

In conclusion, silencing the inner critic is key to healthy eating and fat loss goals. Strategies like positive affirmations, focus on progress, self-compassion, and positive influences can cultivate a constructive mindset, aiding goal achievement.

## V for VOTE

It's easy to dismiss our daily choices as insignificant, but each decision we make is a vote cast for the kind of life we want to live. Just like in a political election, winners don't simply show up and expect success; they strategically campaign and gather support. Similarly, we must actively work towards our wellness goals, making deliberate choices that serve our ambitions.

Navigating the onslaught of messages promoting indulgence or immediate gratification over long-term success can be challenging, especially when they come from loved ones. It's crucial to be aware of these influences and muster the courage to make choices that align with our goals, even when it's tough. This might mean turning down a social event for an early workout or cooking a healthy meal despite feeling tired.

Every decision we make is a vote for the life we aspire to. Each healthy choice builds momentum, confirming our abilities and reinforcing our motivation to stay on course. Every meal, every workout, every prioritized need matters. Like a vote, every choice, no matter how small, shapes the kind of life we lead. Remember, every vote counts towards the life you desire.

# W

## W for WAR

You're in a personal battle against formidable foes: obesity, diabetes, arthrosis, failure, an unhealthy lifestyle, and societal fatphobia. But remember, wars are won one skirmish at a time, and you are capable.

Conquer obesity through incremental diet and exercise changes. Include more fruits and veggies in your diet, engage in daily walks, and increase workout intensity as your fitness improves.

Combat diabetes by controlling sugar intake, consuming nutrient-dense, fibrous foods, and regular exercise to balance blood sugar levels.

To ease arthrosis or joint pain, low-impact exercises like swimming and cycling can help. Foods known to support joint health, such as bone broth and turmeric, can be beneficial.

Failure can seem intimidating when progress is slow, but every step counts. Celebrate small victories and lean on your support system.

Transform unhealthy habits by substituting them with healthier choices. Replace TV-time junk food with carrots or include stretches in long periods of sedentariness.

Lastly, confront societal fatphobia. Learn about its adverse impacts and encourage kindness and respect towards all, regardless of size or shape.

Victory may not come immediately, but tackling each battle progressively will lead to success. Don't hesitate to seek help and remember, you are not alone. You can triumph!

## W for WARRIOR ZONE

I absolutely love the feeling of being in the warrior zone. It's that moment when you push yourself beyond your limits and continue to persevere, even when you should have stopped. It's a moment where you rise above any obstacles and prove to yourself that you are capable of achieving anything you set your mind to. Your body trembles and shakes as it adapts to the new challenge, but you are fueled by your determination and the adrenaline coursing through your veins.

When you finally achieve victory, it's an unparalleled feeling of pride and accomplishment that you carry with you for a lifetime. It's a victory that is yours and yours alone, and one that can never be taken away from you. But, if you're not happy with your current situation, it's likely because you haven't thought about your future self. Instead of making choices that benefit your future self, you've given in to the desires of your present self.

To achieve true success, you have to think about the future and make choices that will benefit your future self. It takes hard work, effort, and dedication, but the rewards are worth it. So don't give up, keep fighting, keep pushing, and strive for that victory that will make your future self proud.

## W for WATER

Water is integral to a healthy diet and promotes fat loss by supporting body functions and preventing dehydration. It curbs appetite as we often confuse thirst with hunger, and regular water intake can mitigate these false hunger signals, aiding in fat loss.

Consuming water can also enhance metabolism, leading to increased calorie burning even during rest. Notably, cold water consumption triggers the body to work harder to achieve body temperature, offering a temporary metabolic spike. Water also supports healthy digestion and waste elimination, crucial elements in a fat loss regimen, by easing constipation and other digestive issues that might interfere with fat loss.

Water helps purge toxins, leading to improved skin health, energy levels, and immune function. But, watch out for sugary and sports drinks loaded with unnecessary calories and sugars, which can impede your fat loss progress. Instead, choose plain or infused water for a healthier, more enjoyable option.

Including high-water-content foods like watermelon, cucumbers, and strawberries in your diet can also support fat loss as they provide water, fiber, and vital nutrients beneficial for overall health. Stay vigilant about signs of dehydration like thirst, dry mouth, and dark urine, and ensure regular water intake.

In conclusion, water is essential for curbing hunger, enhancing metabolism, supporting healthy digestion, and facilitating toxin removal. For successful fat loss and general health, prioritize water consumption and stay aware of dehydration signs.

By following this link, you will find all the tools you need to filter your water:

https://www.the10sprotocol.com/water

## W for WBR WORK BEFORE REWARD

Embarking on a fat loss journey isn't just about weight reduction or improved appearance but rather a lifestyle transformation requiring commitment and dedication. It's essential to temper expectations and understand that lasting fat loss demands a firm commitment to cultivating healthier habits.

To ensure continued success, one must prioritize preliminary work like modifying daily routines, adopting healthier diets, and increasing physical activity. Starting small with sustainable changes is beneficial.

Having a support network is essential, be it friends, family, or professionals such as nutritionists or personal trainers. They provide accountability and motivation, especially in tough times. Surrounding yourself with positive influences also helps maintain focus.

It's crucial to educate oneself about nutrition and exercise, as misinformation is rampant. Researching and consulting reliable sources can safeguard against harmful misguidance.

Alongside habit alterations and knowledge enhancement, fostering a positive mindset is crucial. Despite slow progress and inevitable obstacles, concentrating on positive changes and celebrating small victories can maintain motivation. This positive mindset can counter negative self-talk, benefiting overall health.

Recognize that fat loss is a personal journey. Patience, along with trial and error to discover what works for you, is key. Paying attention to your body's needs is essential.

In conclusion, the essence of fat loss lies in the work before the reward. It's about lifestyle changes, not just diet and exercise. Emphasizing preliminary work, building a support network, self-education, nurturing a positive mindset, and patience are all vital components of a successful fat loss journey, leading to lasting success and a healthier lifestyle.

## W for WEAKNESS

In the journey of fat loss, physical strength is essential but don't underestimate mental resilience. It's critical to recognize and address weaknesses to achieve lasting success.

Often, people struggle with willpower, succumbing to cravings or skipping workouts. However, willpower isn't inborn, but can be nurtured. A strategy like "temptation bundling", which pairs pleasure with a beneficial yet less enjoyable task, can strengthen commitment to healthy habits.

Another common hurdle is lack of self-awareness leading to unhealthy habits. Mindfulness practices like meditation or journaling can increase self-understanding, promoting healthier choices.

Everyone's weaknesses differ; some may struggle with physical limitations or mental health issues that hinder healthy decision-making. Here, professionals like healthcare providers or fitness trainers can help devise personalized strategies.

It's key to treat weaknesses with self-compassion, not criticism. Negative self-talk can hinder progress, whereas recognizing setbacks as part of the process can foster understanding and kindness.

In summary, weaknesses aren't roadblocks but growth opportunities. Identifying and strategizing to overcome them enhances mental resilience. With self-awareness, self-compassion, and openness to new strategies, you can achieve your fat loss goals and enjoy better health.

## W for WEALTH

Physical health and financial prosperity are intrinsically linked. Research suggests that those maintaining a healthy weight often fare better financially than overweight or obese individuals. This connection stems from various factors.

Firstly, physically fit individuals usually have more energy and drive to pursue professional aspirations, which often leads to higher earnings. Good physical health enhances stamina, mental acuity, and overall well-being, resulting in increased productivity.

Secondly, staying fit can translate into financial savings due to lower healthcare costs. Obesity, associated with chronic conditions like diabetes and heart disease, often incurs hefty medical bills. In contrast, fit individuals may face fewer health-related costs.

Thirdly, the healthy habits of fitness-focused individuals, like regular exercise and balanced diets, improve mental clarity and stress management, positively influencing other life domains.

However, while physical health and financial prosperity are interconnected, other factors like education, experience, and skills also impact financial success. Moreover, some fit individuals may struggle financially due to various personal or societal reasons.

Nevertheless, maintaining fitness can bolster financial well-being. Key to this are a balanced diet and regular exercise, combined with support from your network and healthcare professionals. It's essential to approach this journey with patience, persistence, and commitment to sustainable change, laying the foundation for long-term physical and financial success.

## W for WELL-BEING

Diet and well-being are crucial in sustainable fat loss, encompassing both physical and mental health. A balanced diet, filled with whole foods, supplies necessary nutrients, boosts energy, and supports overall health. Similarly, regular physical activity enhances cardiovascular health, reduces stress, and improves sleep quality and flexibility.

Mental health greatly influences our commitment to a fat loss plan. Techniques such as meditation or yoga can help manage stress, reducing emotional eating and boosting resilience. Likewise, adequate sleep, regulating appetite and metabolism, is vital. Chronic sleep deprivation can cause weight gain, so 7-9 hours of sleep a night is recommended.

A robust social support network is also instrumental. Encouragement from loved ones can alleviate stress, bolster motivation, and make sticking to a fat loss plan easier. Friends, family, or support groups can provide invaluable aid on your journey.

Additionally, self-care activities that bring joy and relaxation are crucial in managing stress and promoting overall wellness. Prioritizing self-care can ward off burnout and enhance long-term commitment to fat loss.

In summary, sustainable fat loss goes beyond dieting and exercise, it requires a holistic focus on well-being, including mental health, sleep, social connections, and self-care.

## W for WHAT IS YOUR WHY

Embarking on a fat loss journey is more than just shedding pounds; understanding your personal motivations can guide your path and fuel your commitment. Whether it's for health improvement, a confidence boost, or participating in challenging activities, these reasons can keep you on track amid the journey's difficulties.

Your 'why' not only inspires you but also helps in setting practical, attainable goals. This understanding allows your fat loss journey to cater to your unique needs. For instance, if health improvement is your goal, focusing on nutrient-rich foods becomes crucial.

Recognizing your 'why' also helps foster a healthier relationship with food. Instead of tying fat loss to guilt or self-criticism, it becomes a means of nurturing and caring for your body. This viewpoint guides informed, intentional food choices, focusing on health-boosting foods.

However, gaining this understanding demands introspection and self-reflection, requiring you to assess your fat loss motivations and challenge internalized beliefs about body image and health. Prioritize your health and well-being over societal pressures or unrealistic beauty ideals, allowing for a plan that matches your values and needs, ensuring sustainability.

In essence, understanding your dieting motivations can significantly impact fat loss success and result maintenance. It assists in setting realistic goals, maintaining a positive relationship with food, and making educated food choices. Despite the journey's challenges, considering your personal motivations and goals can illuminate your path towards enduring success. So, before commencing dieting, reflect on your motivations and goals, and let them guide your approach.

## W for WILL

Willpower, the ability to control impulses and delay gratification, is crucial in dieting and targeting fat loss. It's essential for making healthier food choices, sticking to meal plans, and avoiding unnecessary snacking. The omnipresence of dietary temptations, social pressures, and the long-term commitment needed for fat loss often test our willpower.

Despite the challenges, strategies exist to bolster willpower and enhance dietary discipline. Start by setting realistic goals to avoid disappointment from unachievable expectations. Preparation is key; devise meal plans, pack nutritious snacks, and steer clear of temptation-prone situations.

Practice mindfulness, staying present and aware of your cravings and impulses, helping you resist unhealthy temptations. Seek support from friends, family, or online communities to stay motivated and accountable. Reward yourself for your hard work with non-food treats, such as a relaxing massage or a new outfit.

In essence, willpower is a cornerstone of dieting and fat loss success. Strengthening your willpower and cultivating healthy habits make it easier to resist temptations and adhere to your goals. By setting achievable goals, preparing in advance, practicing mindfulness, seeking support, and rewarding yourself, you're paving a successful path in your health journey.

## W for WIN

The first win in a diet for fat loss, be it shedding a few pounds or better fitting clothes, kickstarts a virtuous cycle towards long-term success. Witnessing this initial progress can build momentum and motivation, encouraging consistency in healthy eating and exercise routines.

The beauty of this first win is its power to boost confidence. It shows that your efforts are effective, helping to dispel self-doubt and reinforce your commitment to healthier choices. Moreover, it can help establish healthy habits; consistent progress fosters healthier choices, leading to sustained fat loss and improved health.

Achieving this win calls for effort, dedication, and supportive relationships. Key strategies include setting realistic goals and celebrating even small victories, each contributing to motivation and momentum in your fat loss journey.

Remember, this first win is the beginning of an ongoing journey requiring sustained dedication. Keep a positive outlook, applaud your progress, and use each win as a stepping stone towards long-term success. While it might be challenging, the rewards—enhanced health, boosted energy, and greater confidence—are well worth it. By focusing on positivity, celebrating progress, and leveraging each win, you can ignite a lasting lifestyle change, leading to a healthier, fitter you.

## W for WORK

Undertaking a diet calls for perseverance and commitment, demanding regular exercise and unyielding resolve. While the journey can be challenging at first, your body adapts and you start noticing improvements in your fitness and overall well-being.

One inspiring facet of this journey is the pride from your progress. Every stride mirrors your dedication, bringing a rewarding sense of achievement. Irrespective of your exact goal—running a marathon, improving fitness—each step nudges you closer to success.

Your victories along the way are truly personal triumphs. The joy of reaching the finish line or setting a gym record gives enduring satisfaction and pride. There might be tempting moments, where indulging in a cheat meal seems appealing. However, the gratification from meeting your goals far outshines any temporary pleasure from such indulgences.

By sticking to your diet and investing effort in your goals, you chart your path towards lasting success and a healthier, happier life. Remember, there are no shortcuts, and the work lies squarely on your shoulders. It's your steadfastness and dedication that fuel your success in this journey towards a healthier you.

## W for WORKOUT

Exercise plays a vital role in fat loss, aiding in long-term success. While a healthy diet is key, exercise enhances metabolic rate, muscle building, and overall well-being. Exercise burns calories and fat, helping to create a calorie deficit, crucial for fat loss. Regular workouts also increase muscle mass, improving our metabolism and assisting in maintaining a healthy weight.

Exercise offers more than just fat loss; it promotes overall health. It's been proven to reduce chronic disease risks like heart disease, diabetes, and cancer. Plus, it can positively affect mental health, reduce stress and anxiety, and improve sleep quality.

Incorporating exercise into your fat loss journey needn't be complex or time-consuming. Just 30 minutes of moderate daily exercise, such as brisk walking, jogging, cycling, or strength training, can significantly boost health.

It's key to find a routine that suits you and your lifestyle. Whether you join a gym, take a fitness class, or opt for neighborhood walks or jogs, finding enjoyable, sustainable activities is vital.

In short, exercise is an indispensable part of a fat loss journey. It helps create a calorie deficit, fostering fat loss, and enhances overall health. By integrating regular exercise into your lifestyle and engaging in enjoyable activities, you can achieve lasting success in meeting your fat loss goals.

## W for WORN OUT

Feeling disheartened after unsuccessful fat loss attempts is natural. However, the sheer wealth of accessible information and resources today can equip you for more effective fat loss. The key isn't in quick fixes or fad diets, but sustainable lifestyle changes. While this may sound overwhelming initially, breaking it down into smaller steps makes it achievable. Begin with minor changes, such as incorporating more fruits and veggies into your meals or taking daily walks, to build momentum and confidence for bigger challenges.

Fat loss isn't just about physical health—it involves mental health too. Prioritizing self-care, like ensuring sufficient sleep, indulging in stress-relieving activities like yoga or meditation, and seeking support from loved ones, can enhance your well-being and improve success chances.

The notion of starting might feel daunting, but remember, any forward step is progress. Commitment to the process, belief in your ability to implement positive changes, can lead you to finally achieve your fat loss goals and maintain a healthy lifestyle in the long run. You possess the power to control your health and instigate lasting changes. With this understanding, you can make a fresh start and ultimately attain your fat loss goals permanently.

# X

## X for X-FACTOR

Embarking on a fat loss journey includes picking the right diet, regular exercise, and navigating the X-factor—unexpected events that could offset your progress, such as work stress or sudden illness.

The X-factor can provoke emotional eating, disrupt motivation, and heighten stress, thus affecting your fat loss process. Unexpected events can lead to overeating and feelings of guilt, or stress-induced hormone release, which hampers fat loss.

To counter the X-factor, plan for unpredictable situations. This might involve creating a list of healthy coping mechanisms, like meditation, or determining wholesome comfort food options. Leverage a support network for emotional backing during tough times—this could be friends, family, or professionals.

Setbacks are a regular part of the fat loss journey, and unexpected events are inevitable. But by maintaining a positive mindset, proactively managing the X-factor, and staying resilient, you can stay on track. The X-factor might be a considerable challenge, but with a robust plan, support system, and a positive perspective, you can surmount the X-factor and achieve long-term success. Ultimately, determination, readiness, and persistence make all things possible.

# Y

## Y for YES, IT IS POSSIBLE

Undertaking a fat loss journey necessitates a "Yes, it is possible" mindset. Despite the intimidating nature of fat loss, cultivating a positive attitude significantly influences your progress by overcoming self-doubt and negativity.

Encourage this belief by acknowledging small wins and understanding that fat loss is gradual. Celebrate each achievement, be it losing a pound or feeling healthier. Seek support from those who share your goals to stay motivated, such as support groups, personal trainers, or loved ones.

Set realistic expectations to avoid frustration. Focus on attainable, small goals, such as incorporating more wholesome food into your diet or committing to regular exercise.

Fat loss is more than a number on the scale; it's about adopting a healthy, sustainable lifestyle improving overall well-being, including nutritious eating, sufficient sleep, stress management, and regular physical activity.

Incorporate self-care activities like yoga, reading, or meditation to help maintain focus. Accept setbacks and challenges as part of the journey and see them as opportunities for growth.

In essence, a "Yes, it is possible" mindset is critical in your fat loss journey. With positivity, achievable goals, self-care practices, and supportive connections, you can reach your goals and lead a healthier, happier life. Each step, no matter how small, pushes you forward.

## Y for YO-YO EFFECT

Embarking on a fat loss journey is challenging, especially when facing the yo-yo effect, a frustrating cycle of losing and regaining weight. This cycle, while discouraging, negatively affects physical and emotional health, and understanding it is key to long-term success.

The yo-yo effect slows metabolism. Natural metabolic reduction during fat loss is exacerbated when regaining weight, making subsequent fat loss more challenging and forming a tough cycle to break.

It also impacts muscle mass. Lost weight often includes fat and muscle, but regained weight usually comprises fat, leading to a net loss of muscle over time. This makes maintaining a healthy weight more difficult and harms physical health.

Moreover, the emotional toll from the yo-yo effect can undermine motivation and self-esteem, posing an additional barrier to long-term weight management.

To avoid this effect, prioritize sustainable lifestyle changes over crash diets or extreme exercise. Gradual, sustainable changes help achieve enduring fat loss. Patience and persistence are crucial, as meaningful fat loss requires time. Keep motivated and committed, set realistic goals, and monitor your progress.

A support network of friends, family, or healthcare professionals can provide encouragement, accountability, and guidance, all critical in avoiding the yo-yo effect and achieving lasting fat loss.

In short, understanding the risks of the yo-yo effect and actively avoiding it through sustainable changes, patience, perseverance, and supportive networks can help overcome this challenge, promoting a healthier and happier life. If on a fat loss journey, be mindful of the yo-yo effect and take steps to ensure long-term success.

# Z

## Z for ZERO

ZERO MINUTE

Embarking on a fat loss journey can feel daunting, but the best time to start is now. A "zero minute to wait" mentality emphasizes beginning immediately and focusing on small, immediate positive changes rather than waiting for the "perfect moment". The first step could be as simple as a short walk, swapping a sugary treat for a fruit, or drinking more water.

Progress won't always be linear - there will be ups and downs, but the idea is to keep moving, treating setbacks as learning opportunities, not reasons to give up. Sharing your journey with a friend or family member can help keep you motivated and accountable. Celebrating small victories, tracking progress, and introducing healthy habits like regular exercise, meal planning, and self-care activities such as meditation or journaling into your routine can bolster the "zero minute to wait" approach and lay the foundation for long-term success.

In short, adopting the "zero minute to wait" mindset can kickstart your fat loss journey, leading to a healthier, happier you. Remember, every step counts, so why wait? START NOW.

Finally, you have zero minutes to wait to finally discover the effect of the ABCs of Fat Loss. Enjoy, your healthy lifestyle starts now.

GIVE YOURSELF A ROUND OF APPLAUSE, YOU'VE DESERVED IT.

# CONCLUSION

Congratulations on completing your journey through "The ABCs of Fat Loss." You've embarked on a path that's not just about losing weight; it's about transforming your lifestyle, your habits, and your relationship with your body. As we wrap up this book, let's reflect on the essential lessons learned and the keys to achieving lasting fat loss.

**A is for Awareness:**

Throughout this book, we emphasized the importance of self-awareness in your fat loss journey. Recognizing your goals, understanding your motivations, and being mindful of your eating and exercise habits are the foundation of sustainable change. Remember, self-awareness is an ongoing process, so continue to tune in to your body and emotions as you move forward.

**B is for Balance:**

Balance is the linchpin of successful fat loss. Balancing your diet with nutrient-dense foods, balancing your workouts with rest and recovery, and balancing your mental and emotional well-being are all critical components. Avoid extreme diets and unsustainable exercise routines, as they often lead to burnout and rebound weight gain. Embrace moderation, consistency, and a long-term perspective.

**C is for Consistency:**

Consistency is the secret sauce that transforms intentions into results. It's not about quick fixes but about making small, sustainable changes that you can maintain over time. Whether it's daily exercise, balanced nutrition, or mindful eating, strive for consistency in your habits. Remember that setbacks are part of the journey, but what matters most is getting back on track and moving forward.

**D is for Determination:**

Determination is your driving force, your inner fire that keeps you pushing toward your fat loss goals. It's the mental strength that helps you overcome obstacles and stay committed. Cultivate determination by setting realistic goals, celebrating your successes, and finding inspiration in your progress.

**E is for Education:**

Knowledge is power, especially when it comes to fat loss. The more you understand the science of nutrition, metabolism, and exercise, the better equipped you are to make informed choices. Stay curious and continue to educate yourself about the latest research and trends in fat loss.

**F is for Flexibility:**

Flexibility is the ability to adapt to life's twists and turns while staying on course. Your fat loss journey won't always follow a linear path, and that's okay. Be flexible with your approach, adapt to changing circumstances, and find ways to make healthy choices even when life gets hectic.

**G is for Gratitude:**

In the pursuit of fat loss, it's easy to focus on what you want to change about your body. However, don't forget to appreciate and celebrate your body for what it can do and the progress you've made. Cultivating gratitude can boost your self-esteem and motivation.

**H is for Health:**

Ultimately, fat loss should be about improving your overall health and well-being, not just changing your appearance. Prioritize health by making choices that support your physical, mental, and emotional vitality. Remember that health is a lifelong journey, and fat loss is just one part of it.

**I is for Individuality:**

Recognize that your fat loss journey is unique to you. What works for someone else may not work for you, and that's perfectly normal. Tailor your approach to your specific needs, preferences, and circumstances. Don't compare yourself to others; focus on becoming the best version of yourself.

**J is for Joy:**

Don't forget to find joy in the process. Enjoy the delicious, nutritious foods you eat, savor the feeling of strength and energy after a workout, and relish the sense of accomplishment with each milestone. Fat loss doesn't have to be a joyless endeavor; infuse it with positivity and pleasure.

As you close this book, remember that "The ABCs of Fat Loss" is not an endpoint but a beginning. Your fat loss journey is a lifelong adventure filled with ups and downs, challenges and triumphs. Keep the lessons of awareness, balance, consistency, determination, education, flexibility, gratitude, health, individuality, and joy close to your heart as you continue on this path. Stay committed to your well-being, embrace the process, and trust in your ability to achieve and maintain lasting fat loss. You have the knowledge, the tools, and the inner strength to make it happen. Here's to a healthier, happier you !

# YOU GOT THIS; I KNOW THAT FOR A FACT.

## SPECIAL THANKS

As I come to the end of this book, I am filled with overwhelming gratitude, and I want to take a moment to express my deepest thanks to you. Without you, this journey would not have been possible, and I am incredibly grateful for your presence and support.

I really hope that this book has changed your approach to your diet and your relation with your body and mind.

In case this book has been beneficial for you, I would like you to leave a review on the platform you have bought it from. By leaving a review, it will help this book to be known and maybe help somebody else getting access to the information contents in this book, and maybe change his/her life.

In case you want to know the rest of my work, you can find it on my website www.kalillaichi.com and on my publishing company www.BecomingBetterPublishing.com .

You can also enjoy my others books available on all the platforms:

THE 10S PROTOCOL

TIME THE CURRENCY OF LIFE

THE ABCs OF VITAMINS

# THE 10 "S" PROTOCOL

Discover the secret to long-lasting health and well-being with the revolutionary 10S Protocol! This groundbreaking diet book combines the latest scientific research with practical advice to help you achieve your health goals and transform your life. Dive into this comprehensive guide and explore the ten essential "S" components that will unlock your full health potential:

1. Sleep
2. Stress
3. Sugar
4. Satan's Food vs Superfood
5. Sport
6. Stretching
7. Supplementation
8. S.S.S.B. (Stop Suffocating Start Breathing)
9. Self-Discipline
10. Skin

In The 10S Protocol, you'll learn how to optimize each of these critical components to create a synergistic effect for incredible results. The 10S Protocol is not just another diet fad – it's a holistic approach to health and well-being that is designed to last a lifetime.

Printed in Great Britain
by Amazon